Making shift work tolerable

Making shift work tolerable

Timothy H. Monk, PhD

University of Pittsburgh School of Medicine
Pittsburgh, PA 15213, USA

Simon Folkard, DSc

MRC Social and Applied Psychology Unit
University of Sheffield
Sheffield, S10 2TN, UK

CRC Press
Taylor & Francis Group
Boca Raton London New York

CRC Press is an imprint of the
Taylor & Francis Group, an **informa** business

CRC Press
Taylor & Francis Group
6000 Broken Sound Parkway NW, Suite 300
Boca Raton, FL 33487-2742

First issued in hardback 2018

ISBN 13: 978-1-138-43307-6 (hbk)
ISBN 13: 978-0-85066-822-3 (pbk)

Visit the Taylor & Francis Web site at
http://www.taylorandfrancis.com

and the CRC Press Web site at
http://www.crcpress.com

Library of Congress Cataloging-in-Publication Data

Catalog record is available from the Library of Congress

Contents

Acknowledgements

The authors are grateful for permission to reproduce various figures and tables cited in the text. Grateful thanks are also due to Lisa Crewl, Amy Hayes, Kathy Kennedy and Sandy Christopher at Pittsburgh, where the work was partially supported by funds from the University of Pittsburgh Department of Psychiatry, NIA Grant No AG06836, and NASA Contract No NAS9–18404 to Dr Monk. We also thank Diane Thompson for her work on the manuscript in Sheffield, and Emma Taylor for allowing us to reproduce the transcripts of her interviews with shift workers.

Dedication

This book is dedicated to the affectionate memory of Professor Joseph Rutenfranz who probably did more than any other one person to further the cause of shift work research and improve the shift worker's lot.

Chapter 1

Introduction

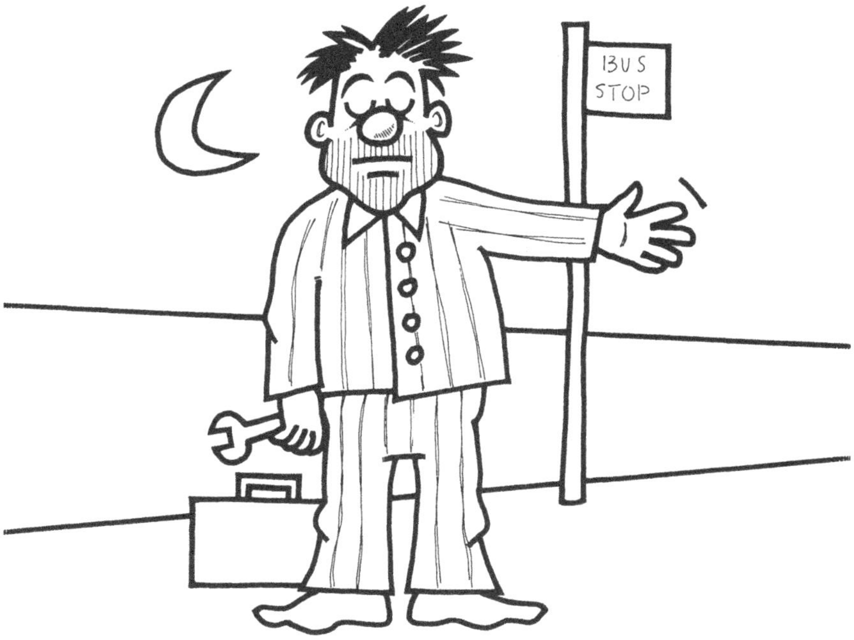

What we mean by shift work

One of the problems we encounter when talking about shift work is that the term means different things to different people. To some people shift work is only really shift work if it involves night work, i.e. work between the hours of 10.30 pm and 6.00 am. For such people, those who only ever work in the evening or the very early morning, or who work split morning and evening shifts, would not come under the category of 'shift workers'. Others have a more comprehensive definition of shift work that includes any regular work that is taken outside the normal 'day work' time window. Then of course there is the problem of whether or not regular overtime comprises shift work, and the problem of defining the outer bounds of the normal day work window.

There are, however, several advantages to the more catholic definition of shift work. Even those who do not have to work at night very often find significant problems in coping with abnormal work hours and in some cases these can actually be worse than those on the night shift. In many cases these problems do not necessarily spring directly from biological causes concerned with the circadian timekeeping system, or the sleep of the individual, but rather from social and domestic pressures that impinge upon their lifestyle and make their shift working routines difficult to cope with (Walker, 1985).

It is for this reason that in this book we shall adopt the broad definition of shift work, defining it as any regularly taken employment outside the day working window, defined arbitrarily as the hours between 7.00 am and 6.00 pm. We shall define any work taken on a regular basis outside that interval as shift work and any individuals involved in that work as shift workers. Thus, we shall include part-timers, full-timers, evening shift workers, early morning shift workers, as well as the rotating and fixed shift workers covered by the more restricted definition.

Some authors suggest that shift work is a relatively new phenomenon which has only come on the scene since the introduction of artificial lighting in the 1800s. They speak of this as having freed us from the tyranny of the sun and talk of a new age and a new frontier where the colonization of the night occurs and we move towards a 24-hour society. In reality, though, shift work has been around for an extremely long time. As Scherrer pointed out in his 1981 historical review (Scherrer, 1981), even in the days of ancient Rome, deliveries of goods were restricted to the night hours to lessen traffic congestion, thus putting most of the delivery sector on to a night shift. In a similar vein, for many centuries the bakers of bread have been toiling through the early hours of the morning in order to have a fresh product available for the day working general public.

The major feature of shift work that has changed through the ages is the number of people who are affected. In the very early days, shift work was, by and large, restricted to a small elite group of particular tradesmen or crafts people who accepted shift work as part of their job. If they were unable to cope with the unusual work hours they simply moved to a different trade or occupation. The main feature of the present industrial age is that there are millions of shift workers who for various reasons find themselves totally unable to move to a day working alternative. It is for the sake of people who are either constitutionally, medically or for social reasons unable to cope with shift work that books like the present one need to be written.

Why do people do shift work?

In both the manufacturing and the service sectors modern society has come to rely upon shift work. Many manufacturing processes either become economically infeasible or are physically impossible without around-the-clock operations. Thus, a nuclear power plant or a glass works simply cannot be shut down at 5.00 in the evening to be reopened at 8.00 am. By their very nature they have to be 24-hour operations. There is also economic pressure towards the introduction of shift work. This pressure takes two forms, the first through the extremely high cost of new machinery and automated processes which very often dictates continuous usage if they are to yield a profit for the company involved. Secondly, there is the response of many employers to fluctuating market places and the high cost of recruiting and hiring personnel. Very often such businesses prefer to require extremely long working hours from their employees than to take the risk of bringing new employees into the company. In both cases shift work is introduced for reasons that are purely economic and which have no relation to the physical attributes of the manufacturing process itself.

In the services sector, shift work has a strong tradition in the medical domain, where nurses and physicians are very often expected either to be on call or actually performing their job on an around-the-clock basis. The areas of policing and transportation also have a strong shift working tradition. There are, however, powerful trends, particularly in the United States, towards quite dramatic increases in around-the-clock availability of various other services. Most notable are the fast food restaurant and grocery industries, which are very rapidly moving towards 24 hours a day, 7 days per week, availability. Again, these changes are ones which are dictated by the market place and/or the absence of legislation, rather than any demonstrable need or attribute of the process involved.

How much shift work is there out there?

Estimates of shift work prevalence vary. In the 1970s the figure most often quoted was 20% of the workforce in both the US (Tasto and Colligan, 1978) and Western Europe (Rutenfranz *et al.*, 1977). Some authors (Czeisler *et al.*, 1985) have since suggested that this is an underestimate. Probably the most accurate figures come from the US census analysis reported by Mellor (1986) which reveals the US shift work prevalence at 22% (16% of full-timers and 47% of part-timers in the workforce), equivalent to about 20 million shift workers. In an analysis of 56,000 Swedish workers, Maurice (reported by Akerstedt and Gillberg, 1982) estimated the frequency at about 30% according to the broadest definition. In the UK, a shift work incidence of 22% was found in a 1968 survey (Anon, 1980).

Kogi (1985) reports an increased prevalence of shift work in developing countries, which often have less restrictive legislation and cheaper labour, thus promoting an export of the practice from industrialized nations.

How is shift work studied?

Shift work is not easy to study. Very often the most important variables are those that occur outside the workplace (e.g. day sleep quality), thus relying to a large extent upon the goodwill of the workers involved. Also, many of the measures are subjective and therefore may be affected by particular predictions (e.g. the move to increase shift pay differentials). There are three basic classes of study, which we shall denote 'field studies','survey studies' and 'laboratory simulations'.

'Field studies' are comparatively rare in international literature because of the high cost and political difficulty of obtaining hard physiological, production and/or subjective measures from a group of workers for a reasonable period of time (e.g. one complete cycle of a rotating shift schedule). Such studies often have a small sample size and require a fairly dedicated group of volunteer subjects (and a tolerant and enlightened management) if circadian rhythm or sleep variables are to be measured properly. When carried out correctly, however, such studies provide an invaluable picture of what is happening to the sleep, circadian rhythms and performance of shift workers under various conditions. Classic field studies are those of Akerstedt (1988) (Sweden), Knauth and Rutenfranz (1976) (West Germany), Tilley and co-workers (1982) (UK) and Reinberg and co-workers (1984) (France). The present authors have also been associated with some limited scale field studies (Folkard *et al.*, 1978, 1979; Folkard and Monk, 1981; Monk and Embrey, 1981; Folkard *et al.*, 1989).

Measures taken in field studies are usually in the circadian, sleep and mood/performance domains. Body temperature is the preferred variable in the circadian domain because of its ease of measurement and stability in indicating the status of the circadian system. Ideally, sleep is measured polygraphically but this is usually impractical (and may actually interfere with normal sleep). Sleep diary measures usually have to suffice. Mood and performance (including subjective activation) are measured by interpolated tests, preferably augmented by measures of actual on-the-job performance.

Survey studies are considerably easier to do, and usually involve the worker in sitting down answering questions during one or two interview or classroom-type sessions, with the data being augmented by personnel, health service and/or absenteeism file searches and a review of production figures. Neither circadian rhythm nor sleep diary measures can be obtained; the best one can usually hope for such variables are questions regarding the *average* timing and quality of sleeps after the various shifts and levels of alertness on them. Survey studies are often carried out before and after an intervention in order to assess its impact. The best known of these is Czeisler and colleagues' 'Potash Mine' study (Czeisler *et al.*, 1982) in which the (positive) effects of several changes, including the speed and direction of rotation of a shift schedule, were assessed. As always, contamination by Hawthorne (placebo) effects can endanger the validity of such studies (Nachreiner *et al.*, 1977).

Laboratory studies attempt to simulate the shift situation in the laboratory. Some use actual shift workers (Walsh *et al.*, 1981) but many are forced to rely upon the conventional 'healthy young men' (Knauth *et al.*, 1978; Weitzman and Kripke, 1981). The major advantage of laboratory studies is that clear and complete recordings of sleep and circadian rhythms (and interpolated mood and performance tests) may be obtained without all of the noise and missing readings that are so characteristic of the field setting. The disadvantages (and they are major) are that social and domestic factors are totally ignored, the individual is not doing a real job, and that the situation only last weeks rather than years. As we shall see when the problems of shift work are discussed, these factors may severely limit the applicability of laboratory study findings. However, laboratory studies may be the only satisfactory way that sleep and circadian rhythms can be accurately measured.

From the preceding discussion it is clear that shift work research does not lie within the boundaries of one discipline, but relies upon the skills of physiologists, psychologists, physicians, sleep researchers and ergonomists amongst others. Teams therefore have to be multidisciplinary, and the results appear in a wide range of sometimes rather obscure journals.

Europe and Japan have benefited from government sponsored independent shift work research groups that were able to give generic findings, published in the open press, and suitable for many different applications. In the United States, most shift work research has been conducted on a consultancy basis by moonlighting academics. As a consequence, many of the US findings remain proprietary and therefore unpublished.

The organization of this book

In writing this book we have drawn upon a variety of sources from a broad range of different countries. While we hope that many of the results are generic and thus appropriate in many different applications, there will inevitably be national idiosyncracies that create problems of generality. Thus, for example, most US food shops are open 24 hours per day, seven days per week, changing the domestic load compared with a European shopper. Similarly, the rapidly rotating schedules favoured in Europe may make certain conclusions (e.g. regarding shift work intolerance and age [Reinberg *et al.*, 1980, 1984]) inappropriate in countries where slower rotating and fixed shift schedules are more common. Thus, in applying the results presented here, the reader must recognize the relative scarcity of the information we can bring to bear, and remember the need for caution when moving them to a specific situation.

What we can be comfortable with is the universality of human biology. We shall see in Chapter 2, that biology is one of the fundamental causes of shift worker problems and, arguably, is also the foundation for the social and domestic problems discussed in Chapter 3. Chapter 4 discusses Colquhoun and Rutenfranz's 'stress and strain' model of shift work coping difficulties as well as our own 'three factor' model of the 'strain' that impinges on the shift worker. Chapters 5 and 6 discuss the health consequences and performance and safety consequences (respectively) of shift work. Chapter 7 covers the 'interindividual differences' between those who seem to be particularly well or poorly predisposed to coping with shift work. The next two chapters of the book deal with solutions. Chapter 8 presents coping strategies for the worker and Chapter 9 strategies for the employer, discussing how one can implement a shift work awareness programme (SWAP) in the company. The book ends with an epilogue, followed by a glossary of terms and definitions and a bibliography listing shift work publications in alphabetical order.

References

Akerstedt, T. (1988) Sleepiness as a consequence of shift work. *Sleep*, **11**, 17–34.

Akerstedt, T. and Gillberg, M. (1982) Displacement of the sleep period and sleep deprivation: Implications for shift work. *Hum. Neurobiol.*, **1**, 163–171.

Anon (1980) Shiftworking: The general picture. In *Studies of Shiftwork*, edited by Colquhoun, W.P. and Rutenfranz, J., pp. 3–15, London: Taylor & Francis.

Colquhoun, W.P. (1971) Circadian variation in mental efficiency. In *Biological rhythms and human performance*, edited by Colquhoun, W.P., pp. 39–107, London: Academic Press.

Czeisler, C.A., Moore-Ede, M.C. and Coleman, R.M. (1982) Rotating shift work schedules that disrupt sleep are improved by applying circadian principles. *Science*, **217**, 460–463.

Czeisler, C.A., Gordon, N.P., Cleary, P.D. and Parker, C.E. (1985) The demographics of shift work: National probability samples indicates US labor force has greater exposure to variable shift work schedules than previously estimated. *Sleep Res.*, **14**, 91.

Folkard, S. and Monk, T.H. (1981) Individual differences in the circadian response to a weekly rotating shift system. In *Night and Shift Work: Biological and Social Aspects*, edited by Reinberg, A., Vieux, N. and Andlauer, P., pp. 365–374, Oxford: Pergamon Press.

Folkard, S., Monk, T.H. and Lobban, M.C. (1978) Short and long-term adjustment of circadian rhythms in 'permanent' night nurses. *Ergonomics*, **21**, 785–799.

Folkard, S., Monk, T.H. and Lobban, M.C. (1979) Towards a predictive test of adjustment to shiftwork. *Ergonomics*, **22**, 79–91.

Folkard, S., Arendt, J. and Clarke, M. (1989) Sleep and mood on a 'weekly' rotating shift system: some preliminary results. In *Shiftwork: Health, Sleep and Performance*, edited by Costa, G., Cesana, G., Kogi, K. and Wedderburn, A., pp. 484–489, Frankfurt: Peter Lang.

Knauth, P. and Rutenfranz, J. (1976) Circadian rhythm of body temperature and re-entrainment at shift change. *Int. Arch. Occup. Environ. Health*, **37**, 125–137.

Knauth, P., Rutenfranz, J., Herrmann, G. and Poppel, S.J. (1978) Re-entrainment of body temperature in experimental shift work studies. *Ergonomics*, **21**, 775–783.

Kogi, K. (1985) Introduction to the problems of shift work. In *Hours of Work – Temporal Factors in Work Scheduling*, edited by Folkard, S. and Monk, T.H., pp. 165–184, New York: John Wiley & Sons.

Mellor, E.F. (1986) Shift work and flexitime: How prevalent are they? *Monthly Labor Review*, **109**, 14–21.

Monk, T.H. and Embrey, D.E. (1981) A field study of circadian rhythms in actual and interpolated task performance. In *Night and Shift Work: Biological and Social Aspects*, edited by Reinberg, A., Vieux, N. and Andlauer, P., pp. 473–480, Oxford: Pergamon Press.

Nachreiner, F., Brand, G., Ernst, G. and Rutenfranz, J. (1977) Zur Kontrolle von Hawthorne-Effekten in

Feldexperimenten. *Z. Arbeitswissenschaft*, **32**, 172–175.

Reinberg, A., Andlauer, P., Guillet, P., Nicolai, A., Vieux, N. and Laporte, A. (1980) Oral temperature, circadian rhythm amplitude, aging and tolerance to shiftwork. *Ergonomics*, **23**, 55–64.

Reinberg, A., Andlauer, P., DePrins, J., Malbecq, W., Vieux, N. and Bourdeleau, P. (1984) Desynchronization of the oral temperature circadian rhythm and intolerance to shift work. *Nature*, **308**, 272–274.

Rutenfranz, J., Colquhoun, W.P., Knauth, P. and Ghata, J.N. (1977) Biomedical and psychosocial aspects of shift work: A review. *Scand. J. Work. Environ. Health*, **3**, 165–182.

Scherrer, J. (1981) Man's work and circadian rhythm through the ages. In *Night and Shift Work: Biological and Social Aspects*, edited by Reinberg, A., Vieux, N. and Andlauer, P., pp. 1–10, Oxford: Pergamon Press.

Tasto, D.L. and Colligan, M.J. (1978) *Health Consequences of Shiftwork, Project URU-4426*, Technical Report, Menlo Park, CA: Stanford Research Institute.

Tilley, A.J., Wilkinson, R.T., Warren, P.S.G., Watson, B. and Drud, M. (1982) The sleep and performance of shift workers. *Hum. Factors*, **24**, 629–641.

Walker, J.M. (1985) Social problems of shift work. In *Hours of Work – Temporal Factors in Work Scheduling*, edited by Folkard, S. and Monk, T.H., pp. 211–225, New York: John Wiley & Sons.

Walsh, J.K., Tepas, D.I. and Moss, P.D. (1981) The EEG sleep of night and rotating shift workers. In *The twenty-four hour workday: Proceedings of a symposium on variations in work-sleep schedules*, edited by Johnson, L.C., Tepas, D.I., Colquhoun, W.P. and Colligan, M.J., pp. 451–465, Cincinnati, OH: Department of Health and Human Services (NIOSH).

Weitzman, E.D. and Kripke, D.F. (1981) Experimental 12-hour shift of the sleep–wake cycle in man: Effects on sleep and physiologic rhythms. In *Variations in work-sleep schedules: Effects on health and performance. Advances in Sleep Research*, Volume 7, edited by Johnson, L.C., Tepas, D.I., Colquhoun, W.P. and Colligan, M.J., pp. 93–110, New York: Spectrum Publications.

Chapter 2

Sleep and the biological clock

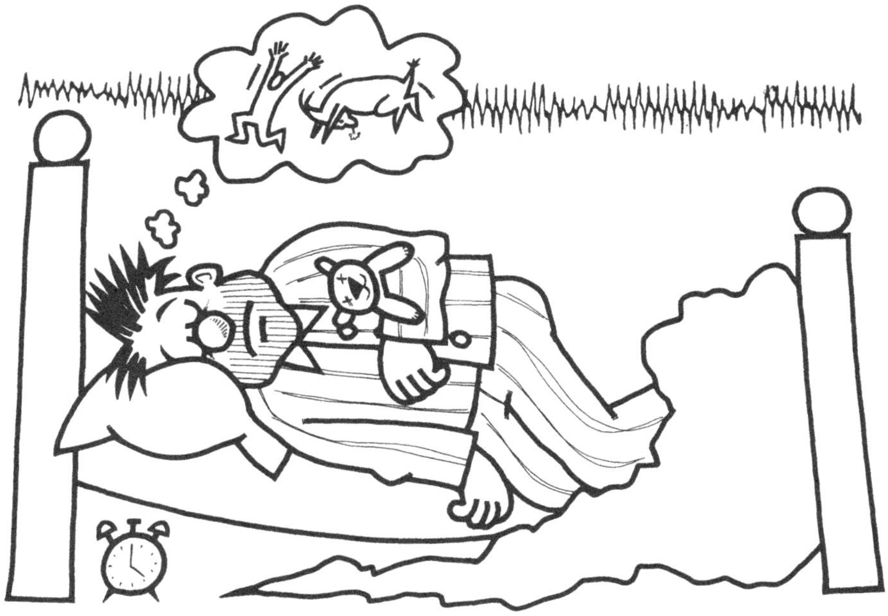

Chronobiology

It is becoming increasingly recognized that like the other creatures on this planet, *Homo sapiens* is essentially a rhythmic species. Cycles with a period of about a day (*circadian rhythms*), less than a day (*ultradian rhythms*), and more than a day (*infradian rhythms*) have all been demonstrated in human physiology and psychology, and undoubtedly comprise a vitally important aspect of the human condition. Clearly, for the shift worker, the dominant periodic domain is that of the circadian rhythms, i.e. those rhythms having a period of about 24 hours.

This chapter is concerned with human circadian rhythms and their relationship to sleep. In understanding the physiological bases of the shift worker's problem it must be recognized that both sleep and circadian rhythms have an important effect, and function in a mutually interactive way.

Human circadian rhythms

Although there has always been a strong folklore about regularity in bedtimes leading to health, wealth and wisdom, the objective study of human circadian rhythms is a comparatively recent development. Not until the 1950s was a scientific investigation of human circadian rhythms begun in earnest and the terms circadian and chronobiology coined (Halberg, 1969). In both medicine and physiology early chronobiologists were continually battling against the prevailing view that homoeostasis led to an utterly constant physiological milieu, and that the circadian rhythms observed by the chronobiologist were at best trivial and at worst suspect. Partly because of this atmosphere of disbelief much of the early work was concerned simply with demonstrating that circadian rhythms do exist, that they are non-trivial in magnitude, and endogenous in origin. Only in the last one or two decades has the discipline really started to define the circadian characteristics of the normal healthy human being and to formulate laws governing the behaviour of that circadian system (Wever, 1979; Aschoff, 1981).

To determine a person's circadian rhythms a particular variable must be measured repeatedly at different points of the day and then the value of that variable plotted as a function of time of day. From this, patterns can be observed showing that there is a systematic change from one time of day to another. One particularly good (and easy to measure) example of this is body temperature. Contrary to popular myth, normal body temperature is not a constant 37°C during the whole day. For day workers, body temperature usually shows a rhythm with a low point at around 5.00 am and a high point around 9.00 pm with a difference of about 0.7°C between the two. Figure 2.1 shows the average daily pattern of body temperature collected in a group of 70 young day workers in a 1968 study by Dr Peter Colquhoun (Colquhoun *et al.*, 1968). This curve is characteristic in showing a comparatively steep rise from early to mid morning, followed by a more gradual rise to the mid evening peak, and then a fairly precipitate decline just prior to bedtime. It is important to recognize that this curve contains not only the rhythm due to the internal biological clock or circadian system but also the changes in temperature that are simply a function of differences in posture and activity. For example, the night readings in Figure 2.1 were taken while the volunteer subjects were in bed and awoken from sleep. Figure 2.2 shows a curve that is fairly similar but is taken from a group of shift workers and comprises only measures taken while the individuals were at work in the control room. This data (taken from Monk and Embrey, 1981) shows that there is still an endogenous rhythmicity present in these individuals even though the 'masking' effect of changes in posture and activity has been balanced out. The day orientation of these rapidly rotating shift workers is evidenced by the fact that both their trough and peak in temperature occurred at the same time of day as the trough observed by Colquhoun in his day workers. However, there is a clear diminution in amplitude resulting from the absence of the 'masking' effect.

Although body temperature has (rightly or wrongly) become the 'gold standard' by which the status of the human circadian system is evaluated, it should be remembered that there is a myriad of other physiological and psychological variables, all showing a consistent circadian rhythmicity (Checkley, 1989). Many of these variables also have a strong endogenous (internally generated) component to them. The most important of these are several hormones which are present in the blood stream and whose presence can also be measured in the urine. The most often cited of these are the rhythms in cortisol which usually peaks in the morning, melatonin which peaks at night, and human growth hormone which peaks soon after sleep onset. Colloquially melatonin can be considered the 'sleep inducing' hormone and cortisol the 'wakening up' hormone, although the exact mechanism of action of these hormones is in fact much more

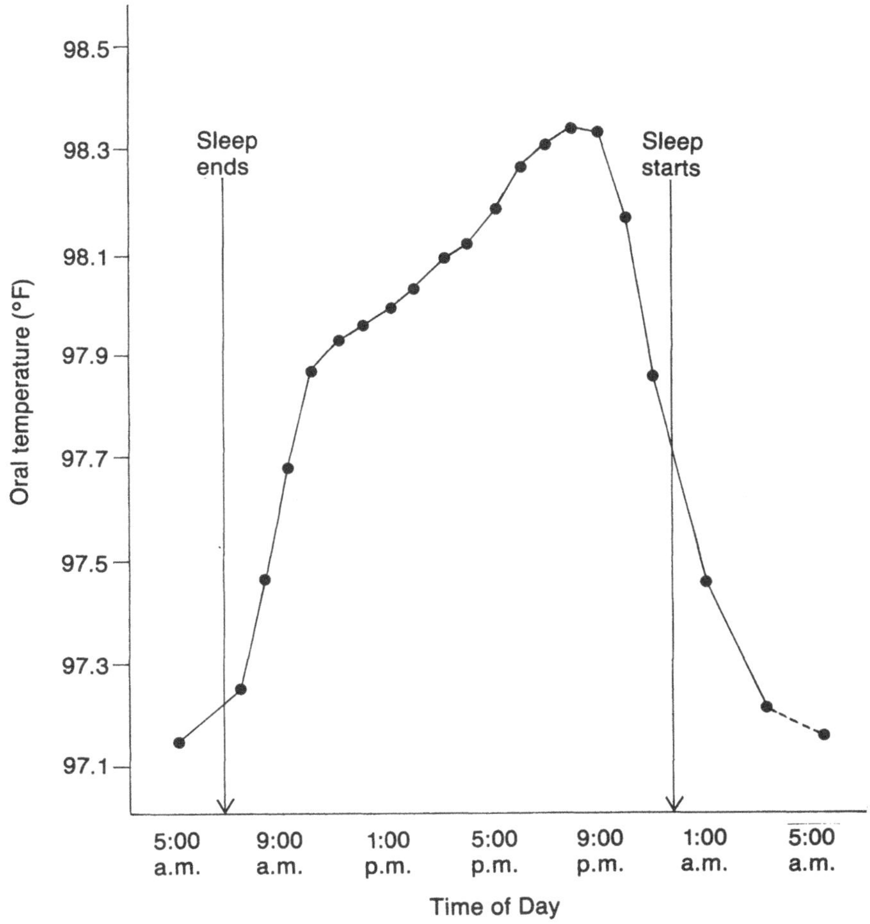

Figure 2.1 Circadian rhythm of oral temperature in a group of 70 young men (after Colquhoun et al.*)*

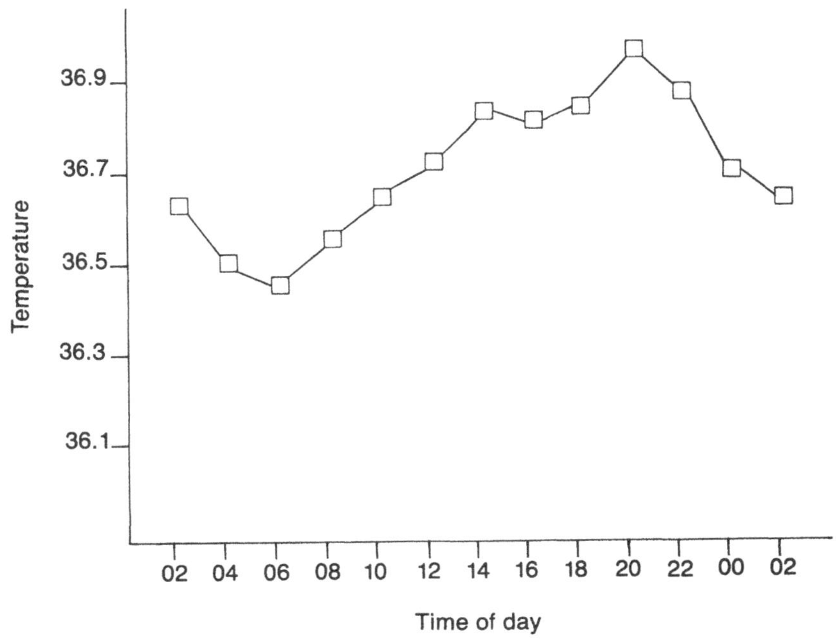

Figure 2.2 Circadian rhythm of oral temperature in a group of six rapidly rotating shift workers studied over a month. Readings were only taken while at work (after Monk and Embrey, 1981).

complicated than this. Arguably, if the blood hormones were as easy to measure as body temperature then it is likely that they would replace temperature as the most often used marker in shift work studies. However, that is not the case; a substantial investment has to be made in both human technical and financial resources if these hormones are to be properly assayed. Very often the researcher uses the more easily obtained measure of body temperature for expedience. Other physiological variables showing a consistent circadian rhythm are heart rate, blood pressure, constituents of the urine (both in terms of electrolytes and in terms of hormones and their metabolites) and also psychophysiological measures such as EEG and Galvanic Skin Response. However, many of these latter rhythms appear to be largely due to sleep/activity, patterning *per se*, rather than more directly to the endogenous circadian 'clock'.

The first, and most important, attribute of the human circadian system is that it is indeed endogenous and self-sustaining, continuing to generate circadian rhythms in mood, performance and physiology even when all external time cues are removed and sleep is suspended. This is illustrated in a study by Froberg (1977) in which 15 young, healthy volunteers were subjected to a 72-hour vigil. During the vigil subjects were sedentary, had no knowledge of clock time and no windows or other time cues to tell them the time of day. They were kept continuously awake and various performance and physiological tests were made. Figure 2.3 illustrates the circadian variation that continued to be present in both subjective alertness and body temperature even though there was no cycling in daylight and darkness or sleep and wakefulness for these 15 subjects, i.e. the circadian system continued to oscillate even when the exogenous (external) factors were

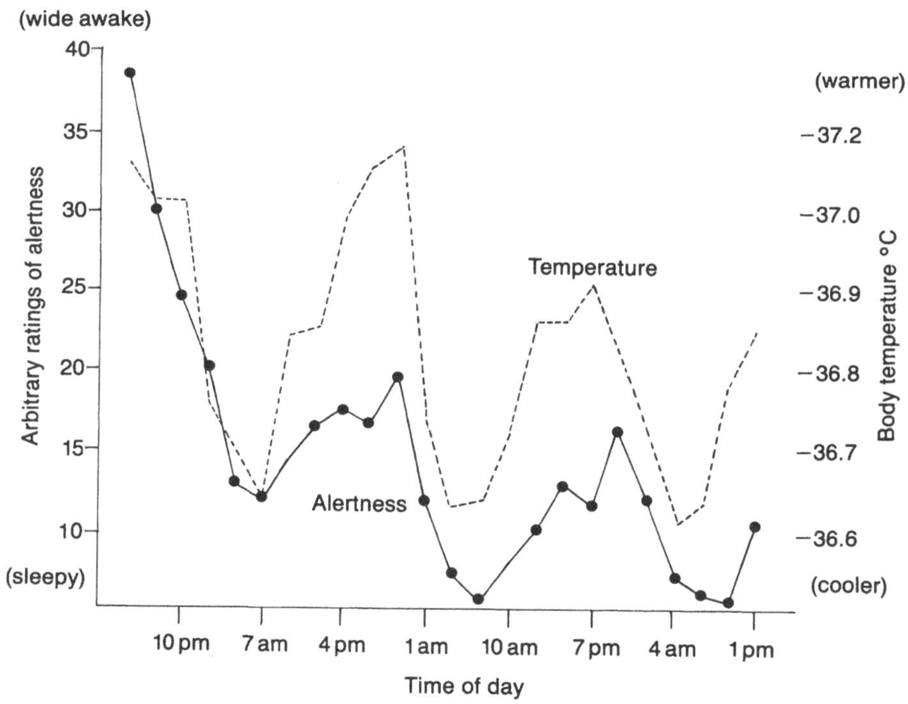

Figure 2.3 Body temperature and alertness from a group of 15 young subjects experiencing 72 hours of constant wakefulness (after Froberg, 1977).

completely constant. Thus, the outputs of the circadian system are not reactions to changes in posture or environment but come from within the individual. In contrast, other measures such as heart rate and noradrenaline (an alerting hormone) showed no persistent circadian rhythmicity under these special conditions, indicating that the rhythms normally found in these measures stem from the cycling of sleep and activity. This important finding has been replicated in many different studies and subject groups.

The second characteristic of the human circadian system, and the one most important for the shift worker, is that much of it is resistant to abrupt changes in schedule. Thus, for example, circadian rhythms in body temperature, cortisol excretion and REM sleep propensity will continue to cycle on an old routine even several days after a new routine has been adopted (Aschoff *et al*., 1975; Weitzman and Kripke, 1981; Klein *et al*., 1972). This results in two adverse consequences for the individual concerned. First, he or she is usually asked to perform at times when the circadian system is calling for sleep and asked to sleep when the circadian system is calling for wakefulness. In the area of transmeridianal flight this is referred to as the 'jet-lag syndrome' (Klein *et al*., 1972). Many regard the inappropriate phasing problem described above to be the main cause of jet-lag. However, there is a second negative consequence of the circadian system's resistance to a change in routine. This can lead to malaise, irritability and gastro-intestinal distress and is caused by a loss of harmony in the various component processes that make up the overall circadian system (Monk, 1987).

A good analogy of the biological clock is that of a symphony conductor on the rostrum making sure that the various instruments are brought in at the right time. After an abrupt shift in routine, it is as if a second conductor mounts the rostrum beating at a different time. Some instruments switch to the new conductor quickly while others take rather longer. Eventually all instruments switch but until that happens the normal harmony is replaced by a cacophony of inappropriately timed events. Within the circadian system there is the need for different component rhythms to ebb and flow at the correct circadian times. Thus, for example, the melatonin rhythm starts to decline as the cortisol rhythm is rising (Figure 2.4). When the abrupt change in routine occurs some circadian rhythms phase adjust more quickly than others. Rhythms such as heart rate that are largely dependent on the sleep/activity cycle adjust relatively quickly, while those that are more dependent on the endogenous circadian 'clock' (e.g. body temperature, melatonin) take considerably longer. Thus, the normal harmony of the overall circadian system is lost and desynchronization occurs (Aschoff *et al*., 1975). The duration of this disharmony depends on both the size and the direction of the change in schedule, but may last several weeks (Weitzman and Kripke, 1981). Both laboratory and field studies have documented decrements in sleep, daytime performance and mood in people who have been subjected to an abrupt shift in routine (Klein *et al*., 1972; Monk *et al*., 1988).

The third characteristic of the healthy circadian system is that it has a natural tendency to run slow. The 'natural' period length of circadian rhythms is determined by isolating people in caves or bunkers where there is no knowledge of either clock time or the daylight/darkness

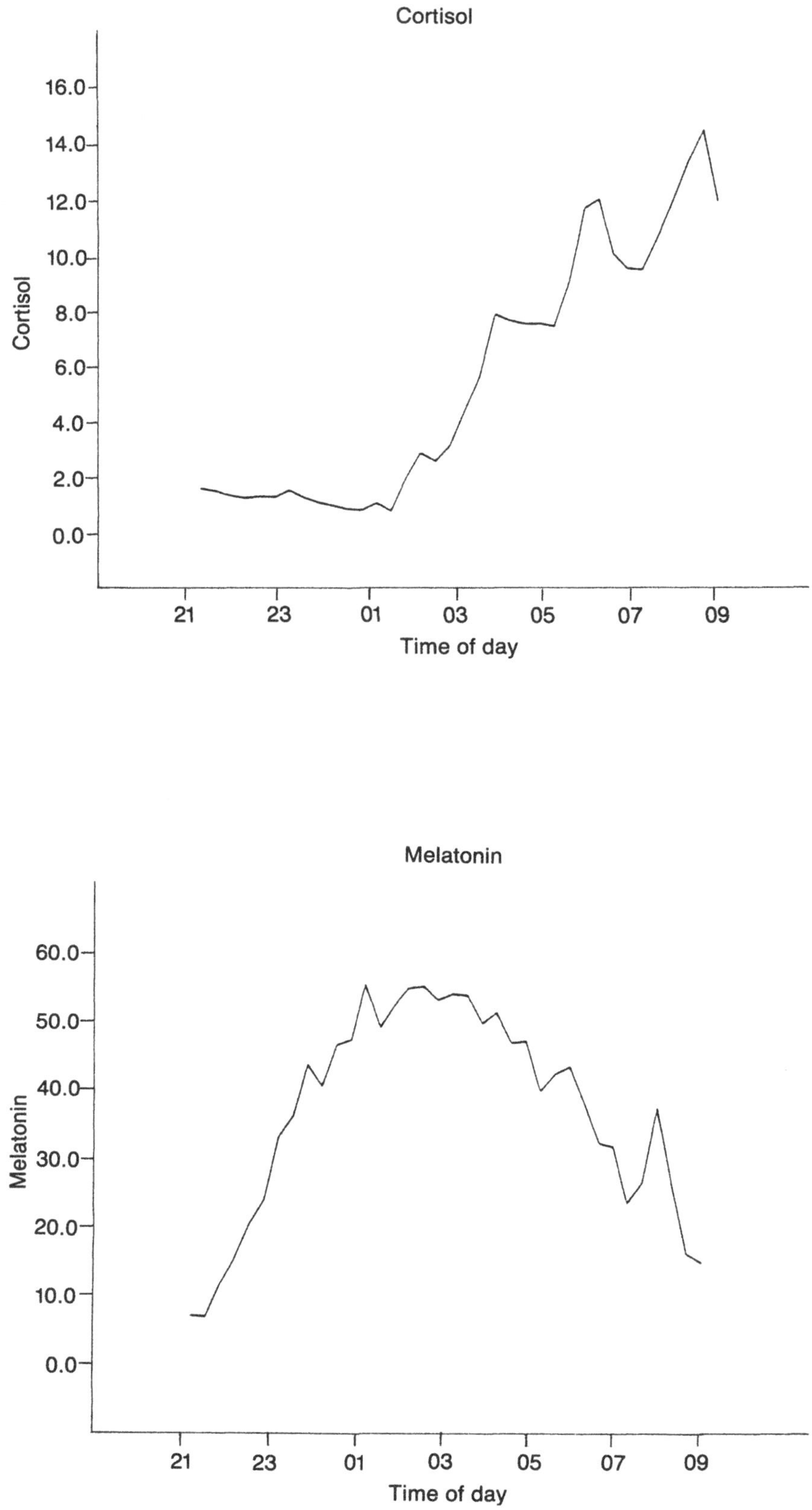

Figure 2.4 Plasma cortisol (microgrammes per 100 ml) and Melatonin (picogrammes per ml) levels from the same group of nine healthy young subjects.

cycle. Subjects are free to go to bed, get up and take meals whenever they like, and the temporal patterning of these events and of the circadian rhythms (e.g. in body temperature) underlying them can be used to glean the period length ('day' length) that is natural to that individual (Wever, 1979). The process is known as *free-running*, and the natural day length often referred to as the *free-running period* or *tau*.

The standard way of illustrating sleep/wake patterns under free-running conditions is referred to as a 'raster plot'. A typical raster plot is shown in Figure 2.5, which is of a young man experiencing four weeks of free-running under temporal isolation (Monk *et al.*, 1985). Time spent in bed (in darkness) is represented by the solid bars. Each day is plotted twice; a total of 48 hours is represented on the x-axis. 'Day of study' is shown on the y-axis. If the free-running day length (tau) was exactly 24.0 hours, then the horizontal bars would line up exactly under each other. The fact that they do not indicates that tau was not 24.0 hours. By fitting a straight line to the beginning of each sleep period we can obtain an estimate of tau, which in this case was 25.0 hours.

In a 'life's work' study of 147 individuals each studied in temporal isolation for about a month, Wever (1979) determined tau for young people to be approximately 25 hours with a standard deviation of 0.5 hours. With increasing age, tau appears to shorten towards 24 hours (Weitzman *et al.*, 1982; Monk, 1989).

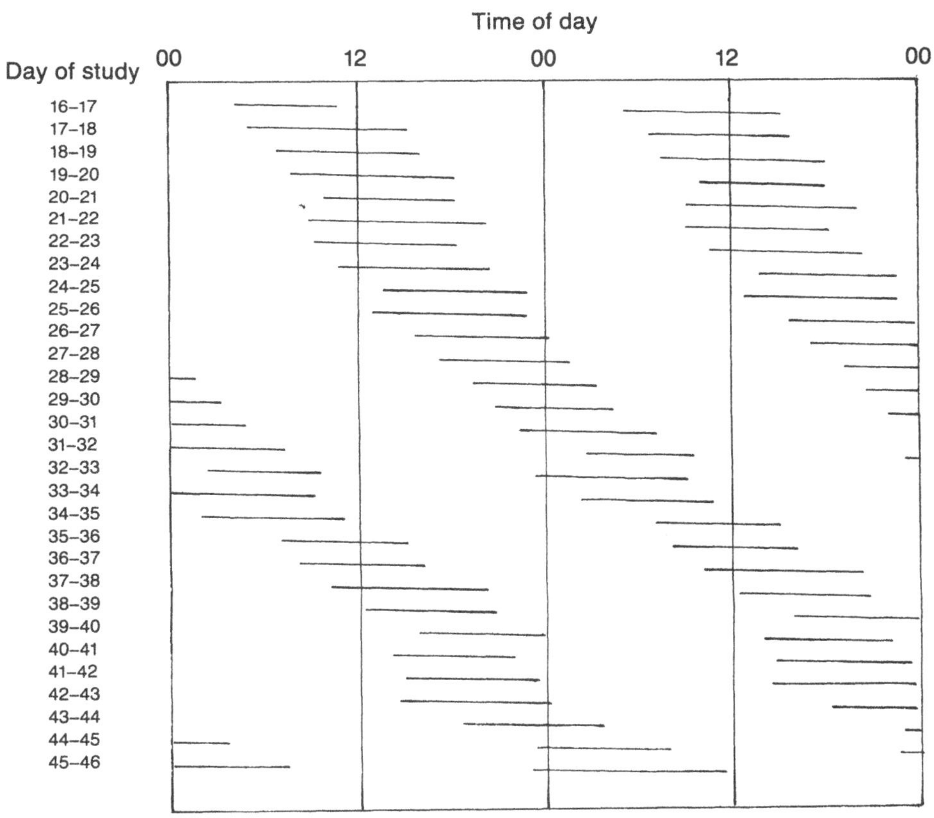

Figure 2.5 Raster plot illustrating the sleep/wake cycle of a 23-year-old male subject experiencing 6 weeks of free-running under temporal isolation. The solid line represents the time spent in bed (in darkness) (after Monk et al., 1985).

Putting these various findings together, it becomes clear that the human circadian system, which usually plays an important role in preparing us mentally and physiologically for sleep, has various properties that are likely to lead to significant problems for the shift worker. The fact that part of the circadian system is endogenous and resistant to change indicates that a move to a night working routine from day working cannot be accomplished biologically in a short period of time. Indeed, as Figure 2.6 shows (from a laboratory study that we carried out in collaboration with Professor Rutenfranz and co-workers at Dortmund) (Monk *et al.*, 1978) the move to a night working schedule may require two weeks of continuous night shifts for the circadian system completely to adjust even in socially isolated subjects. Given the conflicting demands placed on real shift workers by social and domestic factors, the adjustment of their circadian rhythms is likely to be even slower.

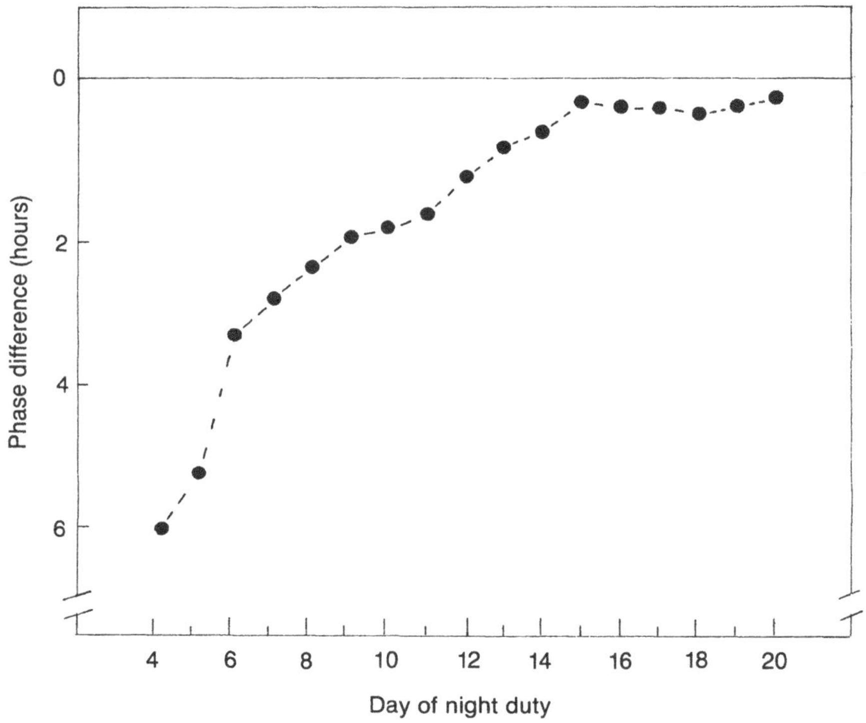

Figure 2.6 The phase adjustment curve (number of hours that a rhythm is 'out of phase' with new routine) for the circadian body temperature rhythm of two subjects working 21 consecutive night shifts (after Monk et al., 1978).

The natural tendency of the human circadian system to run slow suggests that phase delays (to a later timing) are likely to be more easily accomplished by the circadian system than phase advances (to an earlier time), and there is some evidence from both jet-lag (Klein *et al.*, 1972) and shift work (Czeisler *et al.*, 1982) studies to support this. Clearly, one way to try to help the shift worker to cope with the problems stemming from his or her biological clock is to speed up the adjustment process so that the period of disharmony and the period of inappropriate phasing are both reduced to an absolute minimum. As we shall see in later chapters, this requires attention not only to the particular routines or work schedules of the shift worker, but also attention to the time cues (or *zeitgebers*) in the environment that may help or hinder this adjustment process.

Sleep

Like the study of human circadian rhythms, the study of sleep is a relatively new phenomenon with serious objective scientific studies only beginning in the mid 1950s. Even today, many people simply regard sleep as a 'switching off' process leading to a blissful oblivion which is hardly worthy of serious study. Only with the work of Kleitman (1963) and his colleagues in the 1950s was it realized that sleep is indeed a very active process with different forms and depth of sleep observable as the night progresses. Sleep is studied by placing electrodes on an individual's face and head and by measuring the tiny amounts of electricity generated by the brain and facial muscles during sleep. Those changes in voltage are transformed into pen deflections on a polygraph recorder which has a long roll of paper moving through the machine at about half an inch per second. At the end of each sleep session the scientist has about 1000 feet of paper covered in squiggles (Figure 2.7). In trying to make some sense of all these data, sleep researchers have agreed on a classification of particular patterns on the polygraph paper into two main types of sleep, REM and NREM, and four stages of 'depth' of NREM sleep, stages 1, 2, 3 and 4 (Rechtschaffen and Kales, 1968).

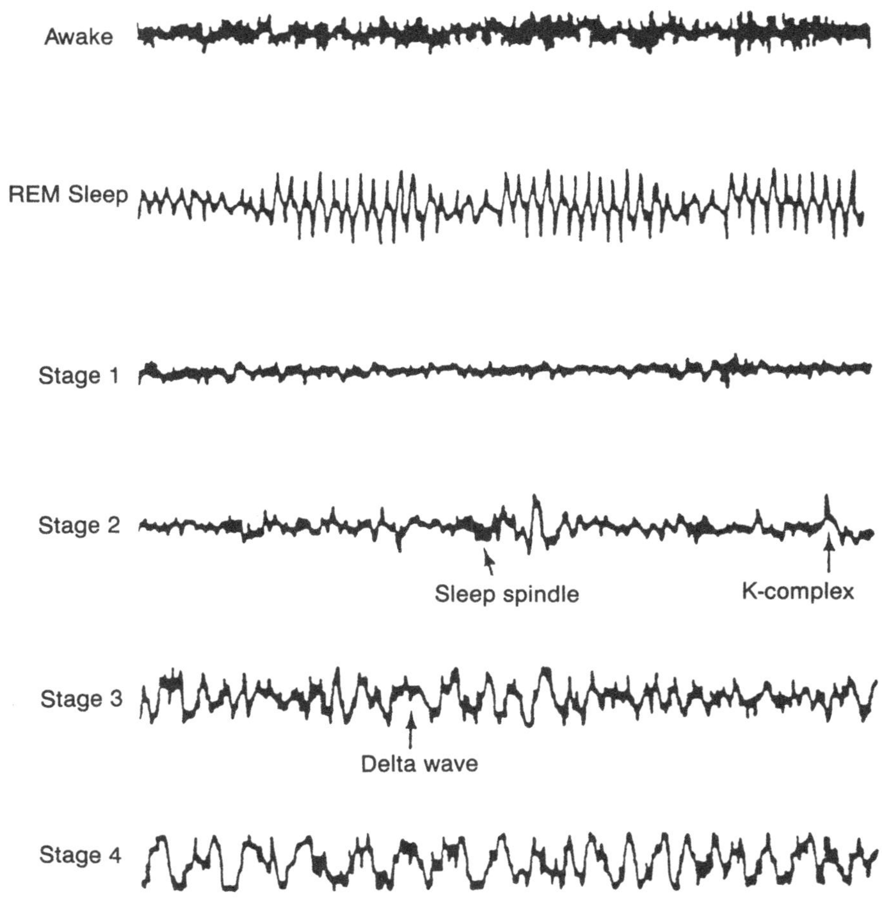

Figure 2.7 Example of a sleep polygraph trace showing brainwave patterns typical of various states and stages of sleep and wakefulness.

REM sleep is very unlike the other sleep stages. The brain wave patterns during REM are much more like those of the awake person and have typical Rapid Eye Movements in which the closed eyes of the sleeping person seem to be scanning quickly back and forth. If an individual is woken up from REM sleep they will probably give a description of a dream, typically the sort of dream that has a story in it. So although people dream occasionally in other stages of sleep, REM sleep seems to be essentially the dreaming form of sleep. REM sleep occurs in regular bursts throughout the night. The patterns start with a burst about 90 minutes after first falling asleep with a new burst of REM appearing every 90 minutes or so thereafter. In a day worker who is normally asleep at night the length of the REM bursts increases as the night progresses, with most REM sleep occurring towards the end of the night. Usually when people wake up spontaneously, either during, or at the end of, the night they do so from REM sleep. This tendency to wake up spontaneously from REM sleep is important to the shift worker because the amount of REM sleep one has is largely determined by the circadian system. Shift workers whose circadian systems are unadjusted are thus likely to have large amounts of REM sleep early on in their day sleeps and this may lead to premature awakenings.

Usually only about 15 to 20% of a night's sleep is REM sleep. We divide the remainder into four different stages or depths. Stages 1 and 2 are very light sleep accounting for about half the night in most middle-aged people (more in the elderly). The two deepest stages (3 and 4) are known as 'slow wave' or 'delta' sleep because of the slow brain waves that they map out on the polygraph paper. Although there is still some debate about what is happening in slow wave sleep, and just exactly why it is important to us, it is becoming increasingly recognized that slow wave sleep is the depth of sleep most important to cognitive restitution and to the restorative aspects of sleep (Horne, 1988). Arguably, it could be concluded that plenty of slow wave sleep will result in an individual feeling well rested in the morning. Fortunately slow wave sleep appears to be primarily determined by length of time awake (need) rather than by rhythmic drives. Thus, the amount of slow wave sleep obtained seems to be more dependent upon how long one has been awake than upon what time of day it is. Indeed, slow wave sleep is the sleep that is first recouped in recovery nights after periods of sleep deprivation. Thus, the categorization of sleep indicates that there are two important types of sleep: REM sleep and slow wave sleep, which have very different properties, and which are going to be differentially affected by shift working routines.

Studies of prolonged partial sleep deprivation both in individuals and in groups has shown that a certain cost has to be paid when people 'short change' themselves on their sleep. There is a cost to be paid both in terms of mood, activation and well being, and also in the ability to perform, particularly in tasks that are inherently boring and monotonous (e.g. driving). Like circadian desynchronization, chronic partial sleep deprivation can lead to symptoms of malaise and fatigue which can significantly impair the productivity and quality of life of the individual. As we have seen before, sleep will inevitably be compromised if the circadian system is not correctly aligned and hence the sleep and circadian system problems of the shift worker are inherently interactive and complementary.

References

Aschoff, J. (1981) (Ed.) *Handbook of Behavioral Neurobiology*, Volume 4, New York: Plenum.

Aschoff, J., Hoffman, K., Pohl, H. and Wever, R.A. (1975) Re-entrainment of circadian rhythms after phase-shifts of the zeitgeber. *Chronobiologia*, **2**, 23–78.

Checkley, S. (1989) The relationship between biological rhythms and the affective disorders. In *Biological Rhythms in Clinical Practice*, edited by Arendt, J., Minors, D.S. and Waterhouse, J.M., pp. 160–183, London: Wright.

Colquhoun, W.P., Blake, M.J.F. and Edwards, R.S. (1968) Experimental studies of shift work. II: Stabilized 8 hour shift systems. *Ergonomics*, **11**, 527–546.

Czeisler, C.A., Moore-Ede, M.C. and Coleman, R.M. (1982) Rotating shift work schedules that disrupt sleep are improved by applying circadian principles. *Science*, **217**, 460–463.

Froberg, J.E. (1977) Twenty-four-hour patterns in human performance, subjective and physiological variables and differences between morning and evening active subjects. *Biol. Psychol.*, **5**, 119–134.

Halberg, F. (1969) Chronobiology. *Annu. Rev. Physiol.*, **31**, 675–725.

Horne, J.A. (1988) *Why We Sleep: the Functions of Sleep in Humans and Other Mammals*, Oxford: Oxford University Press.

Klein, K.E., Wegmann, H.M. and Hunt, B.I. (1972) Desynchronization as a function of body temperature and performance circadian rhythm as a result of outgoing and homecoming transmeridian flights. *Aerospace Med.*, **43**, 119–132.

Kleitman, N. (1963) *Sleep and Wakefulness*, Chicago: University of Chicago Press.

Monk, T.H. (1987) Coping with the stress of jet-lag. *Work and Stress*, **1**, 163–166.

Monk, T.H. (1989) Sleep disorders in the elderly. *Clin. Ger. Med.*, **5**, 331–346.

Monk, T.H. and Embrey, D.E. (1981) A field study of circadian rhythms in actual and interpolated task performance. In *Night and Shift Work: Biological and Social Aspects*, edited by Reinberg, A., Vieux, N. and Andlauer, P., pp. 473–480, Oxford: Pergamon Press.

Monk, T.H., Moline, M.L. and Graeber, R.C. (1988) Inducing jet lag in the laboratory: Patterns of adjustment to an acute shift in routine. *Aviat. Space Environ. Med.*, **59**, 703–710.

Monk, T.H., Knauth, P., Folkard, S. and Rutenfranz, J. (1978) Memory based performance measures in studies of shiftwork. *Ergonomics*, **21**, 819–826.

Monk, T.H., Fookson, J.E., Kream, J., Moline, M.L., Pollak, C.P. and Weitzman, M.B. (1985) Circadian factors during sustained performance: Background and methodology. *Behav. Res. Methods Instrum. Comput.*, **17**, 19–26.

Rechtschaffen, A. and Kales, A.A. (1968) *A Manual of Standardized Terminology, Techniques and Scoring System for Sleep Stages of Human Subjects*, Bethesda, MD: National Institute of Neurological Diseases and Blindness.

Weitzman, E.D. and Kripke, D.F. (1981) Experimental 12-hour shift of the sleep–wake cycle in man: Effects on sleep and physiologic rhythms. In *Variations in Work–Sleep Schedules: Effects on Health and Performance, Advances in Sleep Research*, Volume 7, edited by Johnson, L.C., Tepas, D.I., Colquhoun, W.P. and Colligan, M.J., pp. 93–110, New York: Spectrum Publications.

Weitzman, E.D., Moline, M.L., Czeisler, C.A. and Zimmerman, J.C. (1982) Chronobiology of aging: Temperature, sleep–wake rhythms and entrainment. *Neurobiol. Aging*, **3**, 299–309.

Wever, R.A. (1979) *The Circadian System of Man: Results of Experiments Under Temporal Isolation*, New York: Springer-Verlag.

Chapter 3

Social challenges to the shift worker

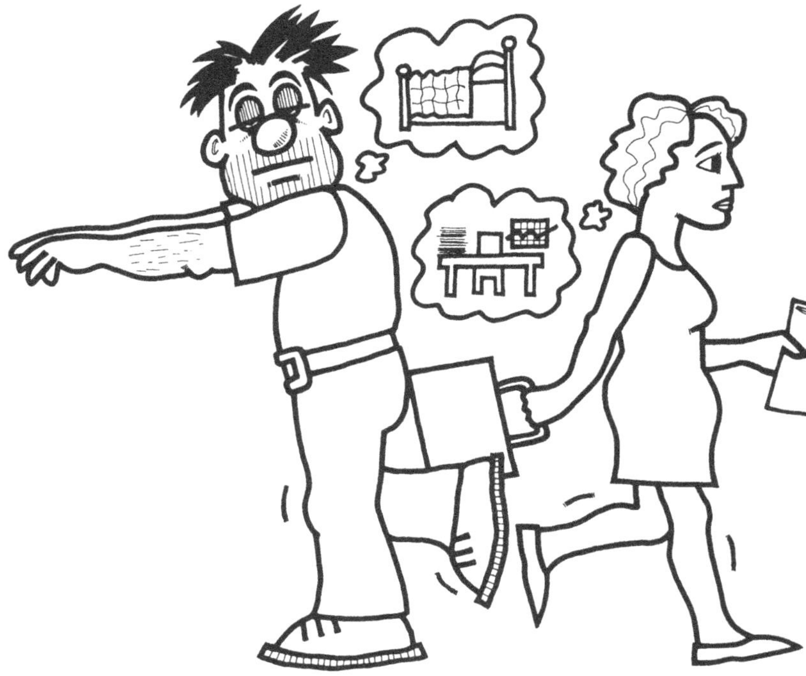

Introduction

As we have seen in Chapter 2 there are sound biological reasons for humans to prefer to take their sleep at night and be awake and active during the day; it is no accident that human society is predominantly a day orientated one, even in modern industrial societies where electric lights have enabled the 24-hour routine to be feasible. Thus, society has quite strong social taboos protecting the night sleep of day workers but has none protecting the day sleep of night workers. For example, few people would even think of calling a friend on a non-urgent matter at 4.00 am but only the most thoughtful and considerate would avoid calling a night worker at 11.00 am: a double standard applies. Society places less value on protecting the day sleep of night workers than it does on protecting the night sleep of the majority. It is almost as if society takes the attitude 'well if you must work at these peculiar times you can't blame us for disturbing your sleep'. It is this permeating attitude, and the biological processes underlying it, that cause much of the tensions to which the shift worker is prone. As we shall see, however, these tensions not only relate to the time the shift worker takes his or her sleep, but also to the intrusions that shift worker schedules make upon time normally set aside for recreation.

Historical perspective

Although the invention of artificial gas and then electric light undoubtedly assisted in the spread of shift work, it did not precipitate it. Shift work has been a part of man's existence for many centuries. As

Scherrer (1981) points out in his historical review of shift work, even in ancient Rome shift work was a part of everyday life. The congestion in the streets of ancient Rome was reduced by requiring that all deliveries be made at night, thus putting the transportation sector onto the night shift. Similarly, soldiers, sailors, watchmen and herdsmen had to accept night work (and other shift work) as a natural and necessary part of their job.

The main difference between the present age and previous times, in regard to shift work, is in the number of people affected, and thus in the opportunities to opt out of shift work. Nowadays there are literally millions of people doing shift work who, if they had the chance, would prefer to do day work. For these people there is effectively no alternative to shift work and it thus behoves society to protect these individuals by legislation, and to assist them in coping through education and the provision of health resources. The recent expansion in the prevalence of shift work has occurred in both the manufacturing and the service sectors of the economy. With the industrial revolution, many manufacturing processes evolved that simply could not be shut down at night since the furnaces and kilns had to remain at the correct temperature. Perhaps more insidious is the economic pressure which can dictate 24-hour operation of plants even when it is not specifically required by the processes involved. With the advent of high technology the machinery required for a particular manufacturing process may be so costly, and depreciate in value so rapidly, that only by operating it 24 hours per day, 7 days a week, can an acceptable financial return be obtained on the investment. Some authors have argued that such reasons for using shift work are unacceptable (Kogi, 1985), but the practice remains widespread. It could be argued, however, that if society is to enjoy the material benefits that our present industrial age has given it then it must also be prepared to pay the price of around-the-clock working.

Shift work in the services sector has enabled a significant improvement to be made in the convenience of everyday life. Although health care has always been available (to a greater or lesser extent) on an around-the-clock basis, other services have only moved outside the 'nine to five' window comparatively recently. In some counties, e.g. the USA, 24-hour shopping has made a dramatic change in people's lifestyles and arguably has encouraged the trend toward dual-income families, and the decline in the number of full-time housewives. This is also true of entertainment and fast food operations which have increasingly provided services outside of the 'normal' time window. It is arguable that in these countries the resultant flexibility in work patterns in those who are part-time shift workers has been a strong positive factor in the trend towards two-income families. Another trend is that of financial need, where, because of increased cost of housing and consumer goods, more than one income is needed to support the household.

A further advantage of shift work in the domestic arena to some families is the child care or older person coverage which it enables. If the husband and wife are on different shifts there is no coverage gap during the day when they are both out to work. Although this might be inadvisable from the point of marital harmony, some workers do quote such arrangements as a significant benefit of shift work and this pattern is undoubtedly one that will continue given the present trends towards dual-income families.

Financial pressures also result in the practice of double jobbing or 'moonlighting' which may be facilitated by shift work. This can either be regarded as an asset (allowing the worker to enhance his or her earning power) or a liability (creating safety, health and productivity concerns as total working hours are increased). Like the babysitting coverage issue, this aspect of shift work is often viewed as an advantage when shift workers are surveyed. Mott *et al.* (1965) found twice as much double jobbing in night workers compared with day workers (23% versus 11%) and Maurice (1975) reported that 33% of continuous shift workers held second jobs. Very often the imposition of a new shift schedule by management (even one that is 'better' from a chronobiological viewpoint) may be resisted by the workforce simply because of its interference with double jobbing schedules.

Increasingly, families need to enhance their income either through double jobbing or through both husband and wife having jobs on either a full-time or part-time basis. Thus, there will undoubtedly be an increase in the grass roots' demand for shift working positions, so that those financial expectations can be met. It is indeed perfectly possible that future employment situations will involve, for a given individual, a whole pot pourri of part-time jobs, filling different temporal niches and different demands on his or her time, rather than a single 40 hours per week traditional job. Interestingly, in Mellor's (1986) review of United States census figures, a full 42% of all shift workers (8.3 million people) were part time, many of them female.

In conclusion it must be recognized that, from an historical perspective, the trend towards ever increasing shift work will be encouraged by three mutually interactive factors: the trend towards costly machinery, the trend towards dual income families (i.e. the absence of a full-time housewife), and the trend towards double jobbing. All three of these influences are likely to increase and feed on each other, producing an ever greater demand for shift work.

The Family

Within the family there are a number of roles that can be adversely affected by the needs of shift work. Problems arise because of the expectations regarding these roles which are carried over from the normal 'five-days-a-week' day working situation. These problems can be just as great for those working the evening shift (where sleep and the circadian system are often minimally affected) as they are for those on the night shift.

Three spouse roles may be affected by shift work, namely, care giver, social companion and sexual partner. The care giver role impinges mainly on the female shift worker who is often faced with societal and family expectations that she should give the same level of 'service' with regard to cooking, clothes mending, cleaning and housework as she would in an exclusively housewife role. Indeed, studies of gender differences in shift work coping have suggested that this societal norm creates many more problems for the female shift worker than do any differences in biology (Gadbois, 1981). However, even biology is working against the female shift worker, since it has been claimed that, on average, females require about 90 minutes more sleep per night than do their male counterparts (Wever, 1979).

Although attention usually focuses mainly on the care giving role of the female shift worker, and the unreasonable expectations regarding this role, there are also care giver roles for the male shift worker that cannot be neglected. Male shift workers often fail to cope satisfactorily in the home maintenance, car maintenance and other 'masculine' care giving roles that he may be expected to fulfil. Alternatively, these roles may preoccupy the shift worker to the detriment of high quality time with his spouse or family, resulting in possibly more family tension than would have arisen had the work been neglected. The social companion role is crucial for many couples, particularly in cultures in which couples meet with other couples on a social basis in the evening and weekends. The absence of a shift worker spouse can cripple not only the shift worker's social life but also that of the spouse.

Finally, there are the problems that shift work creates in the sexual partner role. The day worker comes home from work has a relaxing evening of recreation and then retires to bed with his or her sexual partner. For the night worker the order in which recreation and sleep are taken is usually reversed. He or she typically goes to bed straight after work and usually has recreation in the evening before coming on shift. Thus, the times when the shift worker is in bed and sexually most available are often the times at which lovemaking is either impossible because the spouse is at his or her day working job, or difficult because of the presence of children or other daytime distractions. Moreover, the chronic partial sleep loss experienced by shift workers may mean that lovemaking is simply neglected. Evening shift work can negatively impact on this family role as well, since by the time the evening shift worker goes to bed his or her spouse is very often fast asleep. During a 1985 survey of 1490 workers Tepas (1985) and colleagues showed that more than 70% of those on evening shifts and more than 60% of those on night shift were not satisfied with the amount of time they were able to spend with their spouse, compared with a figure of less than 45% for permanent day workers. It is therefore perhaps not surprising that this study also revealed nearly a 50% increase in divorces for the night working group as compared with day workers, a figure commensurate with that found by Knutsson and colleagues (1986) in a Swedish study. The evidence is not only empirical; one only has to go out and talk to a number of shift workers to conclude fairly convincingly that shift work by and large is bad for a marriage.

Parenting roles are also adversely affected by shift work. For most of the year children are at school, and school is inherently day shift orientated. Thus, for example, evening shift workers may find that they spend a whole week without ever interacting with their children; the children are asleep by the time the shift worker comes home from work and are up and off at school by the time the shift worker wakes up in the late morning (Box 3.1). It is probably because of this that the children of shift workers have been found to do less well at school than those of day workers, especially if both parents are shift workers. In parenting roles, the evening shift worker is probably worse off than the night shift worker. At least the night worker is often able to sleep while the children are at school and to interact with them after school in the early evening before going off to work.

Importantly, negative impacts on spouse and parenting roles not only occur because of the times of day that the individual is required to be at work but also due to the days of the week that the individual must be at work. Society functions under the expectation of a 5-day week, day working, schedule. Very often the fact that the parent is not there

> **Box 3.1**
>
> From a 46-year-old male print room supervisor on rotating shifts. Ninety nights a year. Two teenage children. Wife part-time teacher.
>
> > (My wife) used to leave for work at eight in the morning when I was still in bed and by the time she got home, about four to four-thirty, I went to work. By the time I'd finished at midnight she was in bed, so for six days we would not see each other though we live in the same house. The same went for my kids when they were younger. In the evening when (my wife) gets home on her own, she can't keep the place quiet. She plays music and watches TV and then does not concentrate on watching anything. Just to feel she's someone else with her, more or less.
>
> From a male shift manager of 34. Married with two children, one at school, the other at home. Four-week rapidly rotating cycle with 80 nights a year.
>
> > There are certain days when I do not see [the family] at all, particularly when I go from night shifts to after[noons] on the same day. Because I'm in bed when they are going to school and then I have gone to work by the time they're coming home from school. The following day I only see my son to take to school as I'm back on after[noons] again.

on a Saturday morning for the swimming team meeting, or the soccer game, can be a major handicap for the child involved. Just as there is a definite price to pay for working in the evening and at night, so too is there a price to pay for having to work on a Saturday or Sunday. The nature and comparative values of that price have been evaluated in time budget studies by Knauth and colleagues (1983) and Wedderburn (1967).

The Neighbourhood

As Knauth and Rutenfranz (1975) point out, the neighbourhood can play a major role in creating problems for the shift worker. The most obvious of these is daytime noise, children playing in the street, traffic noise, dustmen and delivery men which can all disrupt the sleep of the night worker. As mentioned earlier, day workers often have an extremely unhelpful attitude towards a shift worker's need for sleep. There are other ways too in which the neighbourhood can have an impact on the shift worker, by expecting his or her participation in events that have been scheduled for the convenience of day workers rather than of shift workers.

Society

Like the family and the neighbourhood, society expects people to work day shifts five days a week and makes life difficult for people when they don't. Evening recreational events, prime time television, sporting events and other society benefits are very often closed to many shift workers because of their unusual work hours. Until the recent availability of domestic VCRs it was impossible for a shift worker to follow a television series or even catch an evening news bulletin.

The interaction between the individual shift worker and society is not an easy one to conceptualize or to study. As Wedderburn (1967) points out, some aspects of a shift worker's interaction with society are made easier by his or her abnormal work routine. Banks and government offices are open during free time, and there is a definite attraction to being at recreation (particularly during the summer months) while others are at work. This, however, may be won at the expense of sleep.

In other respects, though, shift workers are undoubtedly neglected, and feel a certain alienation from society as a whole. The characterization of night work as a frontier is a useful one in this regard. Much as the early pioneers colonized the American West, leaving behind a more comfortable and well supported life in the established East, so the night worker colonizes the night, leaving behind some of the comforts and predictability of day work. Just as the western frontier had a reputation for lawlessness, but a tradition of neighbourliness and mutual help, so too does night work, a trend that was confirmed in an elegant series of studies by Melbin (1978).

References

Gadbois, C. (1981) Women on night shift: Interdependence of sleep and off-the-job activities. In *Night and Shift Work: Biological and Social Aspects*, edited by Reinberg, A., Vieux, N. and Andlauer, P., pp. 223–227, Oxford: Pergamon Press.

Knauth, P. and Rutenfranz, J. (1975) The effects of noise on the sleep of night-workers. In *Experimental Studies of Shift Work*, edited by Colquhoun, P., Folkard, S., Knauth, P. and Rutenfranz, J., pp. 57–65.

Knauth, P., Kiesswetter, E., Ottmann, W., Karvonen, M.J. and Rutenfranz, J. (1983) Time-budget studies of policemen in weekly or swiftly rotating shift systems. *Appl. Ergonomics*, **14** (4), 247–252.

Knutsson, A., Akerstedt, T. and Orth-Gomer, K. (1986) Increased risk of ischaemic heart disease in shift workers. *Lancet*, **12**, 89–92.

Kogi, K. (1985) Introduction to the problems of shift work. In *Hours of Work – Temporal Factors in Work Scheduling*, edited by Folkard, S. and Monk, T.H., pp. 165–184, New York: John Wiley & Sons.

Maurice, M. (1975) *Shift Work*, Geneva: International Labor Office.

Melbin, M. (1978) Night as frontier. *Am. Sociol. Rev.*, **43**, 2–22.

Mellor, E.F. (1986) Shift work and flexitime: How prevalent are they? *Monthly Labor Review*, **109**, 14–21.

Mott, P.E., Mann, F.C., McLoughlin, Q. and Warwick, D. P. (1965) *Shift Work: The Social, Psychological and Physical Consequences*. Ann Arbor: University of Michigan Press.

Scherrer, J. (1981) Man's work and circadian rhythm through the ages. In *Night and Shift Work: Biological and Social Aspects*, edited by Reinberg, A., Vieux, N. and Andlauer, P., pp. 1–10, Oxford: Pergamon Press.

Tepas, D.I. (1985) Flexitime, compressed workweeks and other alternative work schedules. In *Hours of Work – Temporal Factors in Work Scheduling*, edited by Folkard, S. and Monk, T.H., pp. 147–164, New York: John Wiley & Sons.

Wedderburn, A.A.I. (1967) Social factors in satisfaction with swiftly rotating shifts. *Occup. Psychol.*, **41**, 85–107.

Wever, R.A. (1979) In *The Circadian System of Man: Results of Experiments Under Temporal Isolation*, New York: Springer-Verlag.

Chapter 4

Stress and strain

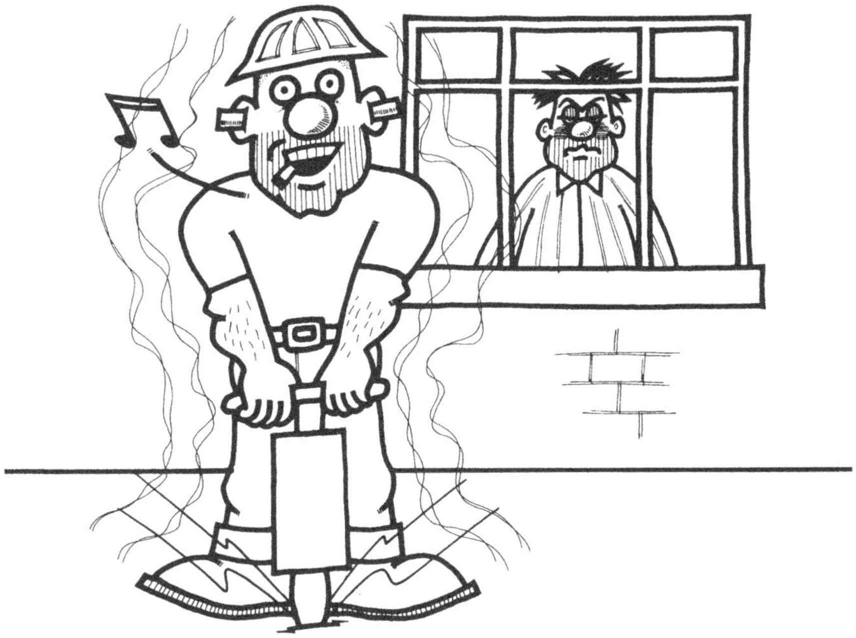

Introduction

From the preceding chapters it is clear that shift work is inherently unnatural to the human being. From both a biological, and hence also a social point of view, we are 'meant' to be day workers. That something is unnatural does not necessarily mean it is harmful of course (centrally heated homes, clothes and antibiotics are hardly 'natural'), but they do indicate a potential for strain in those unable to make the successful transition to a shift working lifestyle. This chapter discusses two conceptual models that are useful in discussing the stresses and strains of the shift worker.

The 'stress and strain' model

In 1980, Colquhoun and Rutenfranz (1980) proposed a 'stress and strain' model of how the various detrimental effects of shift work might arise (Figure 4.1). Broadly stated, this model asserts that such effects do not arise from the actual stress of shift work *per se*, but from the strain that develops within an individual who is trying to cope (more or less successfully) with the unnatural pattern of activity and sleep that shift work may require. Thus, there are intervening variables concerned with coping ability which will determine the level of harm experienced by the individual.

While the distinction between stress and strain may at first seem academic, in reality it is a vitally important one. It implies, for example, that if strain can be reduced (e.g. by the learning of new coping strategies) then even if the stress is the same (i.e., the shift system is

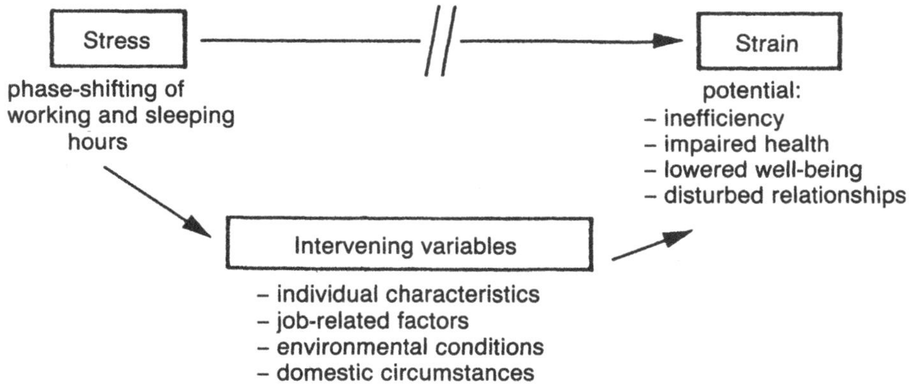

Figure 4.1 The 'stress and strain' model of Colquhoun and Rutenfranz (1980).

unchanged), the level of difficulty (in the safety, health and social/domestic domains) may still be significantly reduced. That is not to say that shift schedules need not be improved (in many cases they most definitely should), but even if they cannot, then education programmes and other countermeasures may still make a difference. Putting it in concrete terms, the incidence of gastric ulcers and heart disease may be as much a function of the social support and educational network given or denied to the shift workers, as it is a function of the precise schedule they work.

Monk (1988) has developed a model to explain how strain arises in the shift worker as a function of three basic areas of stress: circadian system, sleep and social/domestic (Figure 4.2). All three are interrelated, so all three areas must be functioning well for strain to be entirely absent. For example, the circadian system of a night worker

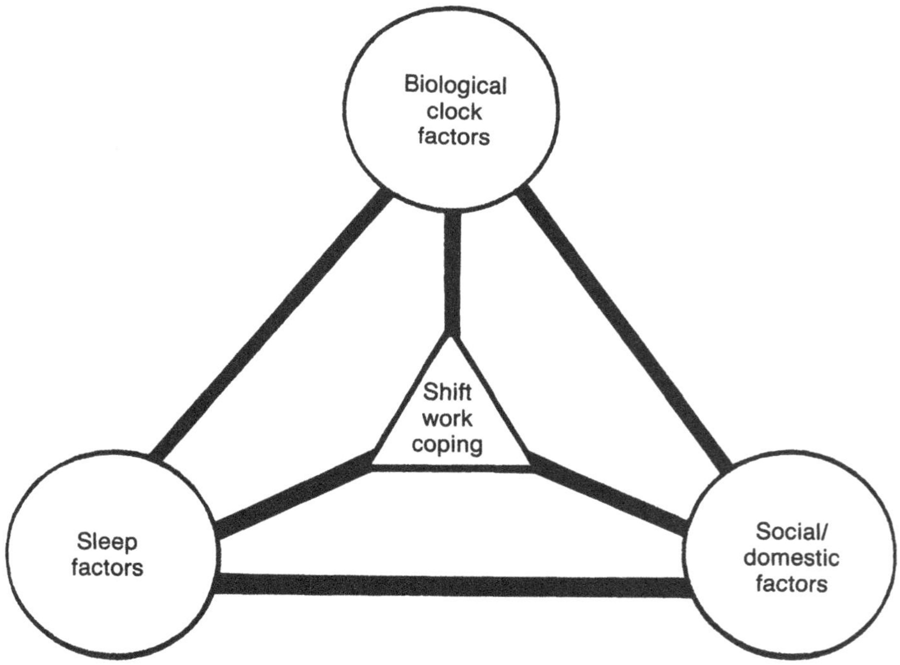

Figure 4.2 A schematic model of the three interactive factors determining shift work strain (after Monk, 1988).

may be successfully re-aligned and the sleep undisturbed, but if these gains are won at the expense of an imminent divorce, then the strain is still there. Most shift workers settle on a compromise between these three components. Sleep may be compromised for time with the kids, circadian adjustment for domestic responsibilities. The aim must be to acquire the balance which involves no critical impairment of any one area.

Strain from the circadian system

As we have seen in Chapter 2, *Homo sapiens* is a diurnal creature with a circadian system designed to expect active wakefulness during daylight and restful sleep at night. The circadian system is kept on track by an entrainment mechanism that uses zeitgebers (German for 'time givers') coming from the environment (daylight/darkness) and the behaviour (social interaction, meal times, etc.) of the individual. The entrainment mechanism is designed to accommodate the one hour or so 'fine tuning' needed to keep the circadian system (whose natural period length is typically closer to 25 hours than to 24 hours) in tune with the 24-hour rotation of the earth (Wever, 1979). As a consequence, the process of adjustment to the abrupt changes in routine occasioned by commencing a run of night work is a slow one, typically taking well over a week (Knauth *et al*., 1981; Weitzman and Kripke, 1981; Monk *et al*., 1988). In addition to the inherent inertia of the circadian system, there are competing zeitgebers (e.g. daylight/ darkness) working to slow down this adjustment process. This is different from jet-lag, for example, where all the zeitgebers encourage adjustment. Many researchers maintain that complete phase adjustment (realignment of timing) very seldom actually occurs, even in permanent night workers.

Apart from the sleep disruption discussed below, there are two major strains placed on the individual by a misaligned circadian system. The first strain arises because of the problem of 'inappropriate phasing'. A major function of the circadian system is to set the stage for sleep at some times of day and wakefulness at others, and a misaligned circadian system will disrupt both sleep and daytime functioning. Sleep will be disrupted by alerting mechanisms such as the cortisol surge and temperature rise. Nightime wakefulness will be impaired by temperature drops and melatonin surges (Akerstedt *et al*., 1982). In some tasks (particularly the monotonous ones such as driving, monitoring and quality control this can cause performance decrements which may severely compromise both productivity and safety (Folkard and Monk, 1979; Monk and Folkard, 1985). Secondly, an inappropriately phased circadian system is in a state of disharmony, akin to the symphony orchestra with its two conductors (Chapter 2). That disharmony can itself result in feelings of malaise and fatigue, as well as certain gastro-intestinal symptoms (Rutenfranz *et al*., 1977; Czeisler *et al*., 1983).

Different circadian strain will therefore be associated with different shift schedules. Ideally, from a circadian point of view, permanent night workers would form a nocturnal sub-culture that maintained a continuous nocturnal orientation to their circadian system by retaining that orientation during their days off. Although this is possible in certain isolated work sites and geographical locations, the overwhelming day orientated time cues (both social and physical) surrounding most night workers in the world make this a largely unrealistic goal. Reversion to a diurnal circadian orientation is all too easy, even during the two or three days of a 'weekend' break (Van Loon, 1963; Monk, 1986). Achieving a nocturnal orientation can be likened to a salmon leaping up a waterfall. It is an arduous process to achieve a nocturnal orientation but all to easy to slip back down to the normal day orientation.

In rotating schedules the strain is also primarily due to the re-entrainment process and to the circadian misalignment that is present until the re-entrainment process is complete. In mid-length rotations such as the weekly ones, complete re-entrainment may never occur, and the worker may find himself or herself in a perpetual state of flux with continuous circadian dysrhythmia, inappropriate circadian re-entrainment and severely impaired sleep and daytime functioning (Tasto and Colligan, 1978).

Rapid rotation accomplishes shift changes in sufficiently rapid succession for circadian dysrhythmia to be absent (the circadian system remains resolutely diurnal), but the strain of inappropriate phasing still remains and may result in severe (albeit short-lived) disruption of sleep and work functioning.

Strain from sleep problems

About 60–70% of shift workers complain of sleep disruption (Rutenfranz *et al.*, 1985). A shift worker's sleep may be disrupted by both endogenous and exogenous factors. Endogenous factors stem from the misaligned circadian system which may fail to prepare the body and mind for sleep and/or wakes the system up (e.g. to eat or use the bathroom) long before 7 or 8 hours of restful sleep have been obtained. Often the worker will complain of being woken by exogenous factors (e.g. traffic noise, children playing) whereas in reality it is his or her misaligned circadian system that is the culprit (Folkard *et al.*, 1979; Akerstedt, 1987).

Exogenous factors may, however, cause severe problems. As mentioned in Chapter 3, the shift worker's day sleep is considered to be much more likely to be disturbed by domestic commitments (shopping, child care, etc.) than is the night sleep of day workers. Households are noisier during the day than at night, and much strain can develop from the chronic partial sleep loss that accrues. Very often, social and domestic disharmony (see below) can develop as the family is blamed for sleep disruptions which may not actually be their fault, but stem, rather, from the shift worker's inappropriately timed circadian system.

Social and domestic strain

The social and domestic strains of the shift worker have been discussed in Chapter 3. Social companion, parenting and sexual partner roles can all be compromised by shift work. Importantly, though, we must remember the interactive nature of the problem. Few of the coping strategies outlined in Chapter 8 will be effective if the social and domestic milieu is not supportive. It is impossible to sleep well if quarrelling with the spouse, or to acquire the correct orientation if the family schedule will not allow it. Also, it should be remembered that evening shift work schedules may be quite benign in their effects on circadian and sleep, but absolutely catastrophic in their impact on family and social life.

References

Akerstedt, T. (1987) Sleep/wake disturbances in working life. *Electroencephalogr. Clin. Neurophysiol.* (Suppl.), **39**, 360–363.

Akerstedt, T., Gillberg, M. and Wetterberg, L. (1982) The circadian covariation of fatigue and urinary melatonin. *Biol. Psychiatry,* **17**, 547–552.

Colquhoun, W.P. and Rutenfranz, J. (1980) Introduction. In *Studies of Shiftwork*, edited by Colquhoun, W.P. and Rutenfranz, J., pp. ix–xi, London: Taylor & Francis.

Czeisler, C.A., Moore-Ede, M.C. and Coleman, R.M. (1983) Resetting circadian clocks: Applications to sleep disorders medicine and occupational health. In *Sleep/Wake Disorders: Natural History, Epidemiology and Long Term Evolution*, edited by Guilleminault, C. and Lugaresi, E., pp. 243–260, New York: Raven.

Folkard, S. and Monk, T.H. (1979) Shiftwork and performance. *Hum. Factors*, **21**, 483–492.

Folkard, S., Monk, T.H. and Lobban, M.C. (1979) Towards a predictive test of adjustment to shiftwork. *Ergonomics*, **22**, 79–91.

Knauth, P., Emde, E., Rutenfranz, J., Kiesswetter, E. and Smith, P.A. (1981) Re-entrainment of body temperature in field studies of shift work. *Int. Arch. Occup. Environ. Health,* **49**, 137–149.

Monk, T.H. (1988) Coping with the stress of shift work. *Work & Stress*, **2**, 169–172.

Monk, T.H. and Folkard, S. (1985) Shiftwork and performance. In *Hours of Work – Temporal Factors in Work Scheduling*, edited by Folkard, S. and Monk, T.H., pp. 239–252, New York: John Wiley & Sons.

Monk, T.H. (1986) Advantages and disadvantages of rapidly rotating shift schedules – a circadian viewpoint. *Human Factors, 28,* 553–557.

Monk, T.H., Moline, M.L. and Graeber, R.C. (1988) Inducing jet lag in the laboratory: Patterns of adjustment to an acute shift in routine. *Aviat. Space Environ. Med.,* **59**, 703–710.

Rutenfranz, J., Haider, M. and Koller, M. (1985) Occupational health measures for nightworkers and shiftworkers. In *Hours of Work – Temporal Factors in Work Scheduling*, edited by Folkard, S. and Monk, T.H., pp. 199–210, New York: John Wiley & Sons.

Rutenfranz, J., Colquhoun, W.P., Knauth, P. and Ghata, J.N. (1977) Biomedical and psychosocial aspects of shift work: A review. *Scand. J. Work. Environ. Health,* **3**, 165–182.

Tasto, D.L. and Colligan, M.J. (1978) *Health Consequences of Shiftwork, Project URU-4426, Technical Report*, Menlo Park, CA: Stanford Research Institute.

Van Loon, J.H. (1963) Diurnal body temperature curves in shift workers. *Ergonomics*, **6**, 267–272.

Weitzman, E.D. and Kripke, D.F. (1981) Experimental 12-hour shift of the sleep–wake cycle in man: Effects on sleep and physiologic rhythms. In *Variations in Work-Sleep Schedules: Effects on Health and Performance, Advances in Sleep Research*, Volume 7, edited by Johnson, L.C., Tepas, D. I., Colquhoun, W. P. and Colligan, M. J., pp. 93–110, New York: Spectrum Publications.

Wever, R.A. (1979) *The Circadian System of Man: Results of Experiments Under Temporal Isolation*, New York: Springer-Verlag.

Chapter 5

Health consequences

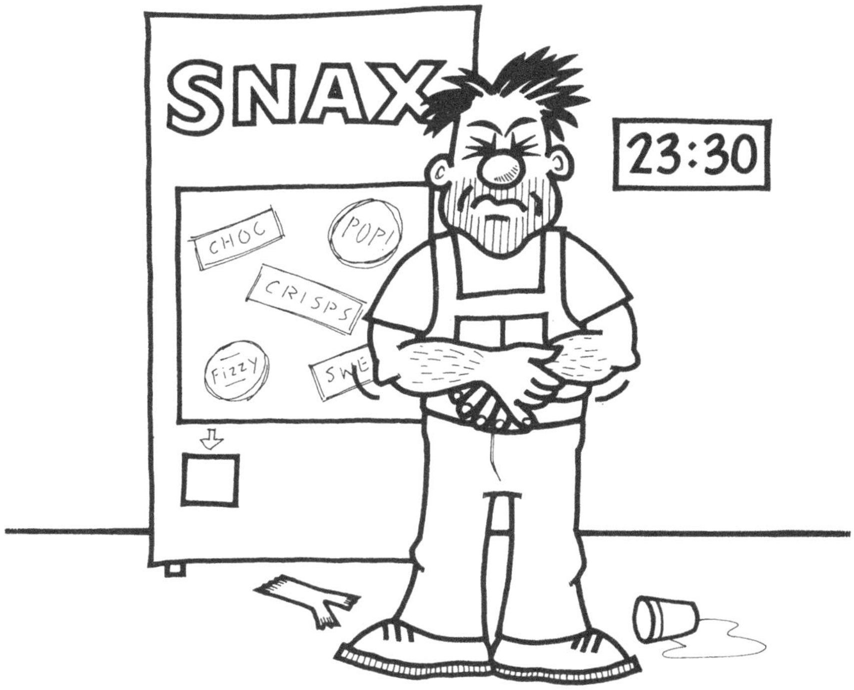

Introduction

A major worry facing shift workers (even those coping fairly well with shift work) is that their health and longevity may be compromised by their shift working routine. Very often shift workers may be resigned to their short-term problems in sleep, sleepiness and other matters, if they can be sure that these discomforts are indeed temporary and that there will be no long-term consequences later on in their life. We are frequently asked when conducting shift work studies in the field or speaking to groups of shift workers, 'Is this shortening my life?' 'Am I going to be ill later on?' 'Am I going to have a heart attack or an ulcer because of it?' Sadly, we are not yet in the position to be able to answer any of these questions with any certainty. Some researchers are renowned for quoting the laboratory simulations of jet-lag on *Drosophila* which reduced the life-span of these insects, but there have been other animal models, most noticeably the mouse, in which rotating shift schedules simulated by changes in the animal's light/dark cycle were actually found to prolong life. So from these animal models the situation is totally unclear.

Unfortunately, when we move to the human studies, there are horrendous methodological and epidemiological problems in answering these relatively simple questions. By and large shift workers are a 'survivor population'. Those who are unable to cope with shift work will, if they can, transfer out and move to day working positions. Thus, particularly in the older age groups, and in the groups with the longest shift working experience, we are presented with a self-selected sample of people who have, perhaps, a constitution that is robust enough to cope well with shift work. Thus, we may be looking not at an average individual with experience of shift work but at the 'superman', as it were, who has been able to survive shift work and may therefore be in the top percentiles of health and robustness. The failure of some researchers to recognize this has led them erroneously to conclude that shift work is not all that harmful. More careful researchers not only look at shift workers and day worker controls, but also look at former shift workers who have transferred out of shift work because they were unable to cope. When we look at these groups we very often see the sequelae of shift work. So in talking about the health consequences of shift work former shift workers should also be included as a group.

The problems outlined above not only affect shift workers' questions regarding their health but also those regarding their longevity. From death certificates or other demographic records, it is very often difficult to find out the extent to which the individual was a shift worker before he or she died. Usually by the time the individual has died they are either retired or have switched to a day working alternative. Moreover, if we compare overall employment categories, for example, comparing trades and professions such as glass making, or steel making which invariably involve shift work, with other manufacturing processes which do not, then the comparison is contaminated by the particular risk factors (e.g. toxins) inherent in the respective workplaces, the stress of the jobs involved, the socio-economic status of the employees as well as differences in geographic location and the surrounding environment.

Notwithstanding all these problems of interpretation we are now fairly confident that there are certain conclusions that we can make about shift work. It should first be stated, however, that these conclusions are primarily with regard to those who do not cope well with shift work. As we have seen in other chapters, many of the social, domestic and circadian rhythm and sleep problems of shift work occur predominantly in those who are failing to cope. So, too, may we conclude that health consequences are more likely to arise in those failing to cope with shift work. This is an important distinction because it means that if we can reduce the strain experienced by the shift worker, for example, by helping him or her with coping strategies, education, and health care provision, then it is possible that the health risk can also be reduced even if the shift work schedule remains essentially the same. For those failing to cope, there is a short, easily remembered slogan regarding shift work and health: 'Shift work is probably bad for the heart, almost certainly bad for the head and definitely bad for the gut'.

The heart

The reason for the word 'probably' in our slogan was that there is still some debate about whether or not shift work is indeed a risk factor for cardiovascular disease. Probably the most authoritative reviewer of health effects in shift work was the late Professor Joseph Rutenfranz (to whose memory this book is dedicated). In reviewing the earlier literature, particularly through the 1960s and 1970s, Prof. Rutenfranz (Rutenfranz *et al.*, 1977) was not convinced that shift work *per se* had any direct effect on either cardiovascular risk factors or on the prevalence of heart disease itself. However, there have recently been some findings from Sweden which quite directly implicate cardiovascular disease as having a higher incidence in shift workers as compared with day worker controls (Knutsson *et al.*, 1986). A 15-year follow-up study of 504 workers in a paper mill plant showed up to double the incidence of heart disease dependent upon the level of exposure to shift work (Figure 5.1). Up to 20 years of shift work experience there was a monotonic rise in cardiovascular disease as a function of shift work experience. After that time, presumably, intolerant shift workers had either died off or switched to day work, and the shift workers then no longer had a higher incidence than the day workers. Clearly, there are alternative explanations for such a finding, related to lifestyle, diet, etc. although some of these factors were taken into account in the Swedish study. Corroborating evidence for a direct effect of shift work comes, however, from a study by Orth-Gomer (1983) who showed that a change in the direction of rotation of shift schedule towards a more chronobiologically sound approach (e.g. a move toward phase delay rotation) directly lowered coronary risk factors such as serum triglycerides. Sleep was also shown to improve. In a less well controlled study, corroborative evidence also comes from a study of Akron city police officers (Ely and Mastardi, 1986), where shift work was shown to be associated with higher norepinephrine levels, thus increasing the risk of ischaemic heart disease.

More evidence needs to be obtained before it can definitively be asserted that shift work is bad for the heart. However, it would seem prudent, simply from the stress aspects alone, to counsel shift workers

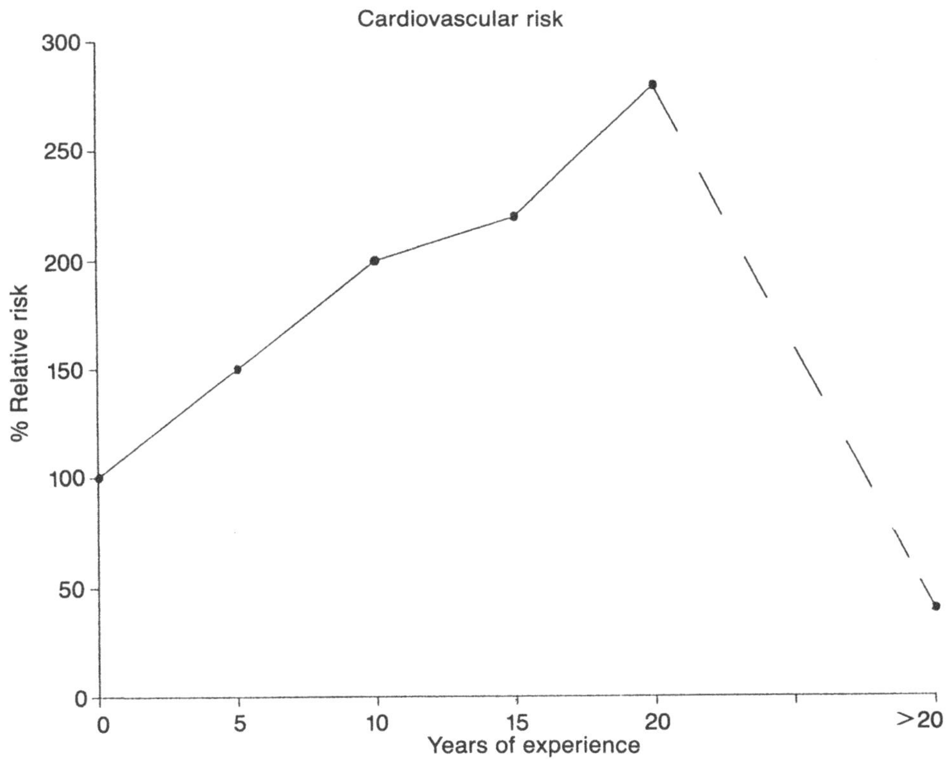

Figure 5.1 Cardiovascular risk rates (Daywork = 100) plotted as a function of years of shift work experience (after Knuttsson et al., 1986).

to avoid behaviours such as smoking, lack of exercise and high lipid diets, that are known to increase the risk of heart disease, since the shift work situation may simply add to the risk. Also, it may eventually be advisable to counsel possible recruits to a shift working position to consider the coronary risk factors associated with their genetic and familiar circumstances, since those too may increase the risk due to shift work. Thus, it may eventually be necessary to suggest that people whose family history includes heart disease should try to avoid employment which requires shift work on a regular basis.

The head

Intuitively it makes sense that shift work is bad for the head. Put someone in a position where they are having very little sleep on a regular basis, their spouse is hostile, their children strangers, and they are permanently punch drunk from 'jet-lag', and it is not really surprising if they become a little nervous and irritable. What we do not yet know is how often that nervousness and irritability can get pushed over the edge into mental illness.

In the USA, much of the circadian rhythm research takes place in departments of psychiatry. The reason for this is that a link has been established between the disease of depression and a dysfunction of the circadian system. Depressed patients show patterns of sleep, early morning awakening and diurnal variations of mood which are very different from those of the healthy individual. At one time it was hoped that many of the symptoms of depression could be alleviated simply by putting the individual on an appropriate circadian routine (Wehr and Goodwin, 1983). Sadly, the initial promise of that simple solution has not been fulfilled, and it looks as though more complex explanations of the circadian dysfunction that occurs in depression must now be considered. However, it remains the case that depression and circadian dysfunction are inextricably linked (Krieger, 1988). Psychiatry is concerned with the direction of causality running from depression to circadian dysfunction. Here, in the shift work situation we are considering the causality in the other direction, namely whether circadian dysfunction can lead to depression. There is, interestingly, some evidence from a study of psychiatric admission to the medical facility at London's Heathrow airport which suggests that that link may indeed be there. Jauhar and Weller (1982) found that depression seems to be associated mostly with passengers arriving after a westward flight and hypomania in patients arriving after an eastward flight. This indicates that, in vulnerable individuals at least, a circadian manipulation can itself induce a recurrence or appearance of psychiatric symptoms.

Unfortunately we do not know, for many of the reasons outlined at the beginning of this chapter, whether or not shift work can be blamed as a risk factor for depression. There is no doubt that shift work can lead to an increase in neurotic type symptoms and to a decrease in well-being and subjective health (Meers *et al*., 1978; Bohle and Tilley, 1989). Unfortunately, there has been no definitive study where strict diagnostic criteria are used to define the symptoms involved. Again, though, it is likely that such a study would founder because of the fact that many shift workers, even showing subclinical symptoms of depression, would simply transfer out and would therefore be lost to the research. A reasonable educated guess is that depressive symptoms are likely to be widespread in a shift working population.

The other side of psychiatric illness which bears upon shift work is that of alcohol and substance abuse. Here again, studies are difficult because of the illegal and potentially job threatening nature of the problem being studied. However, in a survey of several thousand American shift workers, Gordon and colleagues (1986) were able to show an increased incidence in alcohol use, tranquilizer use, and nervousness in rotating shift workers. It seems likely that this study underestimated the prevalence of such problems. In many public transport accidents, concerns about drug and/or alcohol abuse in the shift working driver or pilot has been a definite issue (Lauber and Kayten, 1988). More work is needed but again an educated guess would suggest that alcohol and substance abuse are almost certainly a risk to the shift worker's head.

The gut

There is no question whatsoever that shift work is bad for the gut. Almost every shift worker will complain at some stage or other of 'gut trouble'. This trouble may take the form of increased appetite, decreased appetite, constipation or diarrhoea. It may be as extreme as peptic ulcers or it may be as mild as chronic subclinical indigestion, but the gut trouble is definitely there. This is borne out, too, by empirical studies. Surveys of shift workers invariably show that after sleep problems, gastrointestinal dysfunction comprises a major area in which shift workers (and former shift workers) have more trouble than their day working colleagues (Rutenfranz, *et al.*, 1977) (Box 5.1).

Box 5.1

From a 34-year-old male shift manager married with two children, one at school the other at home. Rapidly rotating cycle, 80 nights per year. At night,

> I would like something that is not a particularly big meal but that is tasty and easy to digest. They do sell that sort of stuff, but they only sell it at mid-day. They cater for the day workers, if you like, for their mid-day meal. But when you work nights, at midnight they only have very basic convenience food and most people go and have cornish pasty and chips and then an hour later they'll come in and say they've got terrible indigestion, or feel sick. But that holds true even if they don't eat. Some people don't eat on nights, they can't. They just don't feel they have any appetite at all on nights. Personally I have, I can eat at nights but I'm pretty choosy about what I have. There are some things I would not attempt to eat like some of the pies, but I might have a jacket potato or something.

Some early reviewers (Harrington, 1978) ascribed this problem to inadequate canteen facilities and/or an inadvisable diet. We feel that although such factors inevitably contribute to the problem, they do not comprise the whole explanation. Common sense tells us that the biological clock must have important interactions with our patterns of eating and voiding. Indeed, one main function of the circadian system is to suppress appetite and the need to void, in order that 7 or 8 hours of restful sleep can be obtained. As Professor Jim Horne (1988) has pointed out, the sleep period is a time of fasting in which stores of food and energy are very definitely depleted. Thus, the circadian system must have the ability to suppress appetite, and to control renal and bowel function for the duration of the sleep episode. Inevitably, therefore, if the circadian system is misaligned, or if it is simply in a state of disarray, the appetite and digestive functions of the individual will be greatly disrupted. In vulnerable individuals this may lead to peptic ulcers. Expert opinion is virtually unanimous in asserting that, apart from the sleep disorders, ulcers and other forms of gastrointestinal dysfunction are the most likely health consequences of shift work.

Because we know that this relationship between gastrointestinal dysfunction and shift work exists, it behoves us to mount a very strong educational drive among shift workers to be sensible about their diet, to consider carefully the timing and the composition of their meals, and to require employers to provide facilities for their shift workers that are equivalent to those they provide for their day workers. Again, we are talking about accumulations of risk. Some of the risk will come from bad diet choices, some from circadian dysfunction while trying to adjust to the changes in routine required by the shift work. Amelioration of the problem should proceed along two fronts, seeking to improve both the circadian adjustment and the meal and food choices that are available to the shift workers themselves.

Conclusions

As we have seen from the work described in this chapter much more research needs to be performed on the health consequences of shift work. It seems probable that when this research is complete, direct health links will be established. The shift working employers of today may find themselves in a similar situation to the asbestos manufacturers of yesterday, living with a legacy of harm which they were unaware of at the time. In the meantime there are certainly educational, shift scheduling and environmental initiatives which the community and employers can, and should, provide in order to lessen at least some of the health risk to which shift workers are exposed on a daily basis.

References

Bohle, P. and Tilley, A.J. (1989) The impact of night work on psychological well-being. *Ergonomics*, **32**, 1089–1100.

Ely, D.L. and Mostardi, R.A. (1986) The effect of recent life events stress, life assets, and temperament pattern on cardiovascular risk factors for Akron city police officers. *J. Human Stress*, **12**, 77–91.

Gordon, N.P., Clearly, P.D., Parker, C.E. and Czeisler, C.A. (1986) The prevalence and health impact of shiftwork. *Am. J. Public Health*, **76**, 1225–1228.

Harrington, J.M. (1978) *Shiftwork and Health. A Critical Review of the Literature*, London: HMSO.

Horne, J.A. (1988) Why We Sleep: the Functions of Sleep in Humans and Other Mammals, Oxford: Oxford University Press.

Jauhar, P. and Weller, M.P.I. (1982) Psychiatric morbidity and time zone changes: A study of patients from Heathrow Airport. *Br. J. Psychiatry*, **140**, 231–235.

Knutsson, A., Akerstedt, T. and Orth-Gomer, K. (1986) Increased risk of ischaemic heart disease in shift workers. *Lancet*, **12**, 89–92.

Krieger, D.T. (1988) Abnormalities in circadian periodicity in depression. In *Biological Rhythms and Mental Disorders*, edited by Kupfer, D.J., Monk, T.H. and Barchas, J.D., pp. 177–196, New York: The Guilford Press.

Lauber, J.K. and Kayten, P.J. (1988) Keynote Address: Sleepiness, circadian dysrhythmia, and fatigue in transportation system accidents, *Sleep*, **11**, 503–512.

Meers, A., Maasen, A. and Verhaegen, P. (1978) Subjective health after six months and after four years of shift work. *Ergonomics*, **21**, 857–861.

Monk, T.H. (1988) *How to Make Shift Work Safe and Productive*, Des Plaines, Ill. American Society of Safety Engineers.

Orth-Gomer, K. (1983) Intervention on coronary risk factors by adapting a shift work schedule to biologic rhythmicity. *Psychosom. Med.*, **45**, 407–415.

Rutenfranz, J., Colquhoun, W.P., Knauth, P. and Ghata, J.N. (1977) Biomedical and psychosocial aspects of shift work: A review. *Scand. J. Work. Environ. Health*, **3**, 165–182.

Wehr, T.A. and Goodwin, F.K. (1983) Biological rhythms in manic–depressive illness. In *Circadian Rhythms in Psychiatry*, edited by Wehr, T.A. and Goodwin, F.K., pp. 129–184, Pacific Grove, CA: The Boxwood Press.

Chapter 6

Performance and safety consequences

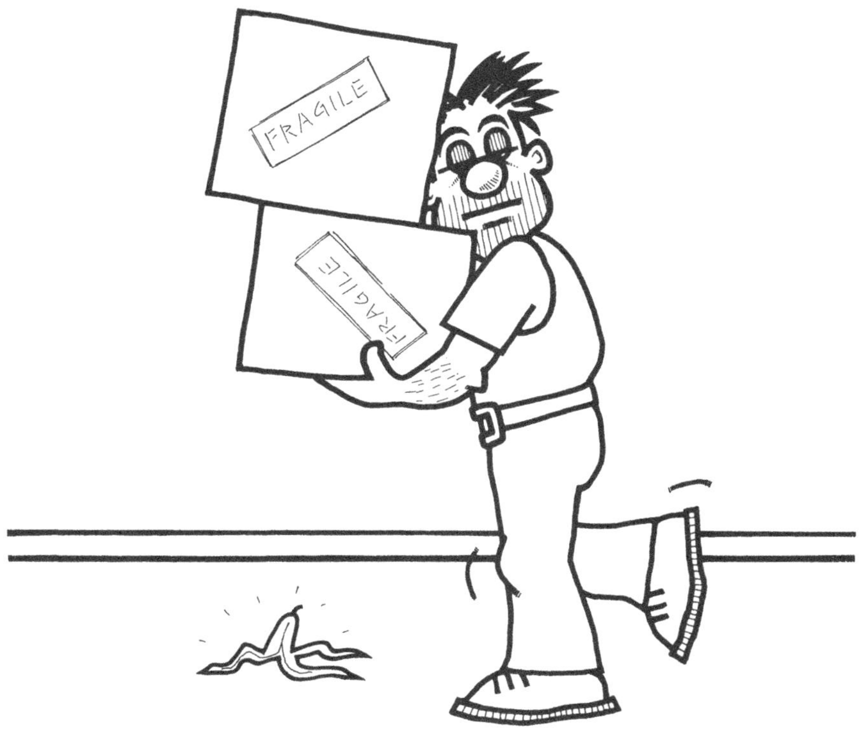

Introduction

As anyone who has lived with young children can attest, performance, mood and alertness are all impaired when one has to attend to a task in the middle of the night and with insufficient sleep. It would, indeed, be very surprising if performance and safety were not compromised by shift work. As this chapter demonstrates, though, these issues are much more complicated than initial impressions might indicate. Performance and safety issues must sometimes be separated, and must be considered in terms of both the sleep loss and the circadian aspects of the problem.

Shift worker safety

While there are occasionally greater environmental risks associated with shift work than with day work, e.g. because of no daylight, or increased chemical exposure on 12-hour shifts (Brief and Scala, 1986), these are usually outweighed by the reduction in the number of people around, i.e. 'human traffic'. Indeed, when the accident rate is not expressed as a percentage of 'traffic load', the number of accidents is often fewer on the night shift than on the other shifts (Wojtczak-Jaroszowa and Jarosz, 1987). However, when accidents are expressed in terms of rate per worker on the job, the night shift often comes out worst (DeVries-Griever *et al.*, 1987). This illustrates the point that it is primarily the unadjusted shift worker who is the agent of risk, rather than the environment around the worker.

One of the most frequently quoted industrial accidents is the Three

Mile Island incident which threatened a whole community and crippled an entire industry. This incident can be traced to human errors committed by weary shift working controllers mid-way through the graveyard (or night) shift (Ehret, 1981). Other accidents have a similar aetiology and abnormal hours of work and circadian dysfunction can often be blamed (Lauber and Kayten, 1988).

There are a number of different ways in which maladjusted shift workers can become agents of risk to themselves and others. The first way is through sleepiness at work (Akerstedt, 1988), the aetiology of which was discussed earlier. Sleepiness at work can lead to the problem of missed signals (e.g. a red light, a dial going critical), or of inappropriate responses to correctly perceived signals (e.g. landing an airplane on the wrong runway) as well as that of actually dozing off to sleep on the job. These effects are also important in the journey to and from work.

Although it is tempting to regard all dangerous shift workers as being overly sleepy, there are groups of maladjusted shift workers who are not sleepy at all, but who may be just as dangerous. These workers are too upset and angry to be sleepy, either for biological reasons (circadian dysfunction, sleep loss) or social ones (an imminent divorce). Such mood changes can lead to a cavalier or directly aggressive attitude towards the handling of dangerous machinery, and to the absence of concern for the safety of those around them.

The third means by which shift workers can become agents of risk is through simple performance decrements. Although not subjectively sleepy, workers may be suffering performance decrements which (e.g. in the meat packing industry) may lead to personal injury because of the critical nature of the work being undertaken.

Thus for safety, as was the case for health, the conern is particularly with those shift workers who are not coping well for one reason or another. Measures that either reduce the stress on the shift worker (e.g. by the adoption of more benign schedules) or the resulting strain (e.g. support systems and education) will undoubtedly improve safety both at the workplace and on the journey to and from it.

Performance and safety consequences of shift work

While safety and performance are inextricably linked, it is quite possible for performance efficiency (and thus productivity and competitiveness) to be impaired without any additional safety risk necessarily occurring. Shift work performance, however, is a very complex issue. This complexity stems not only from the influence of task demands on both time-of-day effects in performance efficiency and the oscillatory control underlying them, but also from the influence of sleep deprivation effects, subjective and objective health effects, motivation effects (which will be influenced by social and family problems), and the effects of interindividual differences on both normal rhythm parameters, and the rate at which such parameters readjust to a change in routine.

Although it represents something of an oversimplification, our earlier conceptual model (Folkard and Monk, 1979), which is illustrated in Figure 6.1, represents a useful framework in which to consider these effects. Essentially, this model (like the later one of DeVries-Griever and Meijman [1987]) reinforces the point that the 'on-shift' performance of the shift worker is the product of many different factors, some interacting directly, others having their effect through changes in the adjustment process.

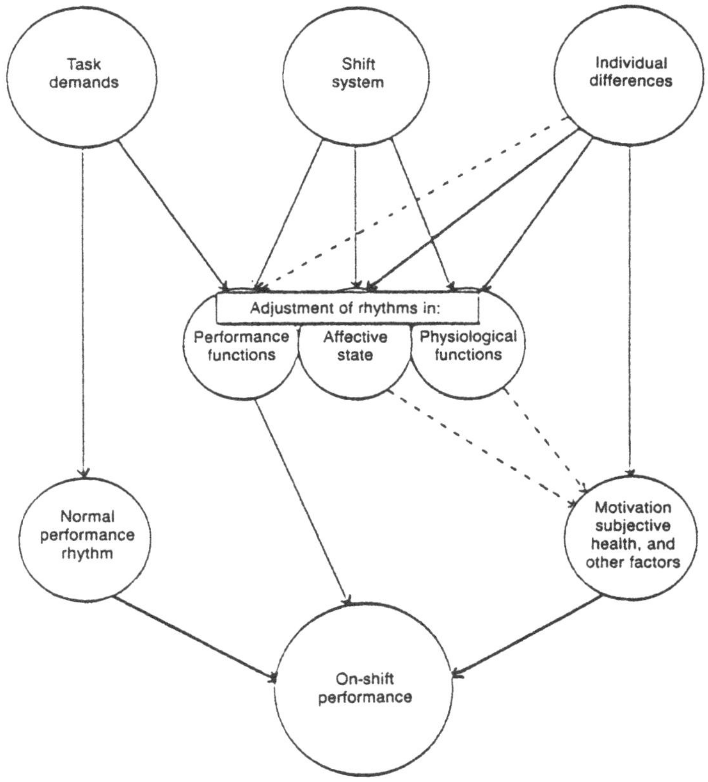

Figure 6.1 A conceptual model of the factors affecting 'on shift' performance. Solid lines represent known influences, and dashed lines probable ones (after Folkard and Monk, 1979).

The three major inputs to the system are task demands (i.e. the levels of vigilance, physical and cognitive work required of the individual), the particular shift system used (very different effects spring from fixed (permanent) shifts than from rotating schedules, for example), and interindividual differences (including the worker's personality, age, health, sleep needs and behaviour patterns) (Moog, 1987). These factors will then serve to affect the adjustment process in performance function (circadian performance rhythms), affective state (circadian rhythms in subjective vigilance, mood and well-being) and physiological functions (sleep being the most crucial, but also the circadian rhythms in temperature and neuroendocrine function). The interaction of those adjustment effects will then influence the worker's on shift performance, both directly and through indirect effects on his or her subjective health and well-being. Thus, it cannot simply be asserted that a night shift performance will be poor because the worker is then 'at a low ebb'. That assertion may be quite wrong for some tasks (Monk and Embrey, 1981), and is certainly remiss in leaving out the sleep deprivation, health and motivational effects that can often outweigh the strictly circadian ones (DeVries-Griever and Meijman, 1987).

There are major problems in trying to determine intershift differences on 'real task' performance. The most important of these is the difference in working environments. Not only lighting levels, but also supervision levels, group morale and distractions can all be very different indeed between night shifts and day shifts (Monk and Folkard, 1985). Also, poorer performance can occur on the night shift simply because there is nobody there to repair broken machines (Meers, 1975). Not only the work environment, but the work itself may be quite different on the night shift. Very often particular parts of the job are actually saved for the night shift, either because the process demands it (preparing things for shipment in the morning), or to make life easier for the night workers (e.g. long-running computer jobs held back in order to be run at night). Even in continuous-process operations, complicated development work may intrude during the day, but not at night (DeVries-Griever and Meijman, 1987).

Despite all these problems and complications, there are a few studies that have been able to obtain relatively continuous 24-hour 'real task' data, and indeed these studies show a remarkable similarity

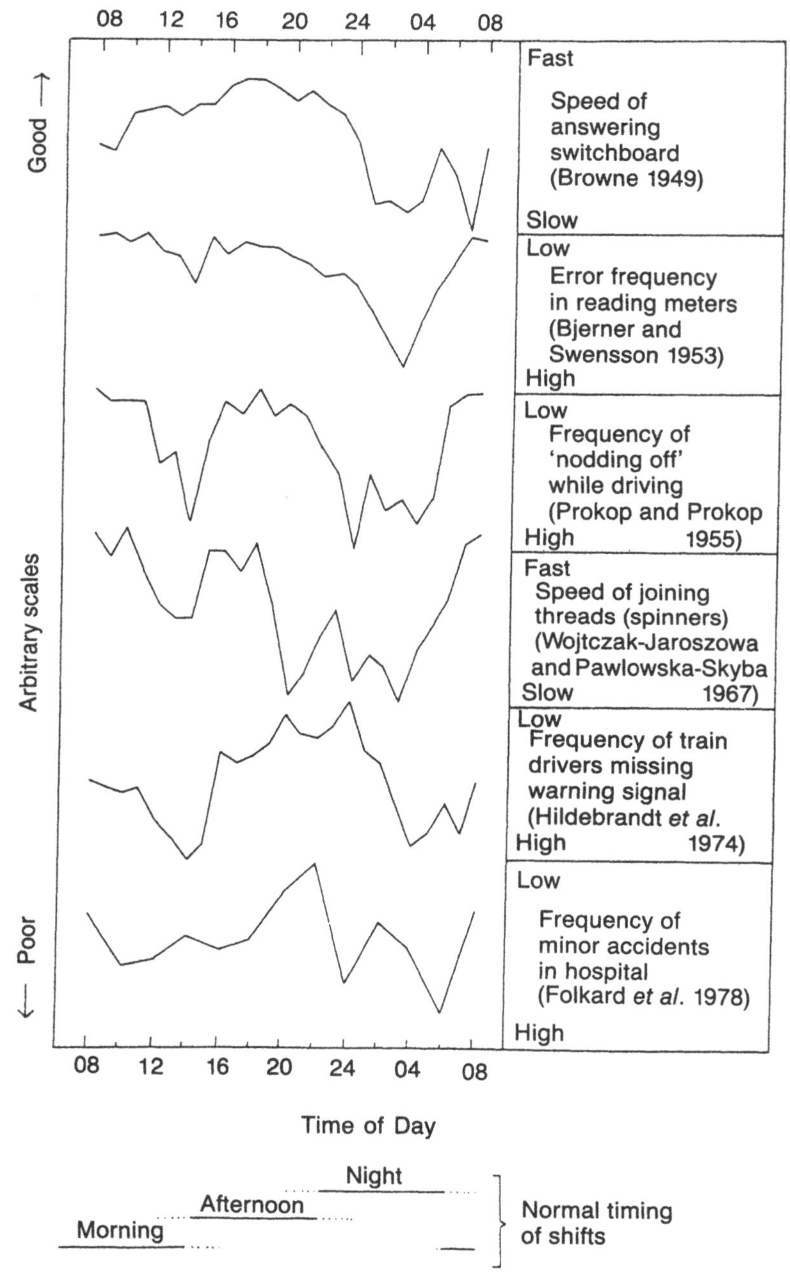

Figure 6.2 Variations in job performance over the 24-hour period (after Folkard and Monk, 1979).

in time-of-day function (Figure 6.2). The six studies can be divided into three that actually measure the speed (Browne, 1949; Wojtczak-Jaroszowa and Pawlowska-Skyba, 1967) or accuracy (Bjerner and Swensson, 1953) with which the primary task is done, and three that measure the consequences of lapses in attention or vigilance (Prokop and Prokop, 1955; Hildebrandt *et al.*, 1974; Folkard *et al.*, 1978). All six are in agreement in showing performance to be worse during the night hours, although in three of them there is also evidence of a pronounced post-lunch dip of almost equivalent magnitude. In Hamelin's recent study (1987) of truck drivers the risk of accident from midnight to 2 am was found to be more than double the normal average.

Thus, it would seem reasonable to assert that, in general, night shift performance (and, indeed, very early morning performance) is inferior to normal day shift performance. However, as we have been careful to point out, there are a number of different ways in which night shift performance can be degraded, not all of them directly circadian. Additionally, it is possible that differences in motivation level can differentially affect time-of-day functions. Khaleque and Verhaegen (1981) showed this in a comparison of cigar-making speeds between morning and afternoon shifts; significantly, time-of-day differences only appeared in highly stressed workers who were making considerable efforts to gain extra piecework bonuses. Thus, it is possible that circadian effects are only evident when workers are under pressure. In the absence of such pressure, night workers may be able to equate day shift and night shift performances because both are considerably suboptimal. In that case, overall intershift differences in productivity are more likely to occur from absenteeism and tardiness effects than from individual performance *per se* (Fischer, 1986; Farrell and Stamm, 1988).

Circadian studies

An example of a field study using an interpolated task is provided by Wojtczak-Jaroszowa and colleagues (1978) who administrated three very brief (1-minute) performance tests to ten shift workers on rotating morning, afternoon and night shifts. The tests measured manual dexterity, and simple and complex serial search performance, and were given just before the start of the shift, and again after 4 and 8 hours of work. All three tests showed the night shift to have the worst performance. For the manual dexterity and simple serial search tasks, the morning and afternoon shift performance levels were roughly comparable, but for the more complex serial search task the morning shift was clearly the better of the two. All three shifts showed declines that were equivalent in magnitude to the circadian effects.

Sleep deprivation studies

Although all studies of shift workers' performance must have circadian rhythms as a major area of interest, some studies have tended to focus on the sleep deprivation aspects rather than the more strictly circadian ones. One of these is the 'work–sleep study' carried out by Professor Don Tepas and his associates (1981a, b) in Chicago. This comprehensive study brought actual shift workers into the sleep laboratory for polysomnography and performance testing while they continued to work, commuting from the laboratory rather than from home. Tepas' team used a vigilance task presented just prior to bedtime, and a machine paced additions test at bedtime and upon awakening.

The subjects comprised ten night workers, ten day workers and ten (slowly) rotating shift workers who were working day or evening shifts at the time of study. Night shift workers were the group that performed worst on all three performance tests (there being no reliable differences between the other two groups). The performance differences were not accompanied by any equivalent differences in body temperature, but were correlated with the polysomnographic data in a way that was typical of a subject undergoing chronic partial sleep deprivation.

Rather than bringing shift workers into the laboratory for polysomnography and performance assessment, Tilley and colleagues (1982) took the tests out to the field. Twelve shift workers were studied for one complete cycle of their weekly rotating shift system. The results were very similar to those found by Tepas' group with day sleeps appearing to be disrupted and of shorter duration than night sleeps. As would be predicted from circadian considerations, reaction speeds (both simple and multiple choice) were slower on the night shift. However, there was also strong evidence for a night-to-night deterioration in performance, which the authors interpreted in terms of a build-up of partial sleep deprivation. They concluded that rapid rotation of shifts, with shorter runs of night duty, might be more conducive to better sleep and performance.

Supervision levels

Anyone who has been a shift worker will attest to the freedom and relaxed attitudes that can occur during the absence of day working management. Some shift workers can abuse that freedom, sleeping on the job, abusing drugs, shirking or performing non-job activities (e.g. running a card school). Productivity in those situations will inevitably suffer and it would be foolish not to address that issue before embarking upon some elaborate chronobiological intervention. The other side of the coin, though, is that many shift workers positively enjoy the lack of supervision, and given the proper motivation might be highly productive given the 'esprit de corps' that night shift work often engenders.

Overall hazards to worker and public

In conclusion, it must be realized that not only the worker, but also his or her family, and indeed the surrounding community, face hazards to their safety and well-being as a result of shift work. In evaluating these hazards the multifaceted nature of the shift work issue must be recognized. At one extreme, there may be rare but highly significant events such as a near meltdown at a power plant, a chemical plant explosion or a train derailment. These highly visible events can affect (and indeed threaten) thousands of lives and have a massive effect on the well-being of surrounding communities. At the other end of the spectrum are the comparatively frequent events such as vehicular accidents on the drive home from work and minor injuries at work. Because of their lower profile in the news media these events may tend to be relatively ignored. In financial terms (and, indeed overall human misery) it is quite possible, however, that the sum total of the frequent small events is as important to society as that of the occasional dramatic ones. Both are often the result of shift worker errors, and both should be taken into account when society evaluates the cost-effectiveness of shift work.

References

Akerstedt, T. (1988) Sleepiness as a consequence of shift work. *Sleep*, **11**, 17–34.

Bjerner, B. and Swensson, A. (1953) Shiftwork and rhythm. *Acta Med. Scand.*, **278**, 102–107.

Brief, R.S. and Scala, R.A. (1986) Occupational health aspects of unusual work schedules – A review of Exxon's experiences. *Am. Ind. Hyg. Assoc. J.*, **47**, 199–202.

Browne, R.C. (1949) The day and night performance of the tele-printer switchboard operators, *Occup. Psychol.*, **23**, 121–126.

DeVries-Griever, A.H.G. and Meijman, T.F. (1987) The impact of abnormal hours of work on various modes of information processing: A process model on human costs of performance. *Ergonomics*, **30**, 1287–1299.

Ehret, C.F. (1981) New approaches to chronohygiene for the shift worker in the nuclear power industry. In *Night and Shift Work: Biological and Social Aspects*, edited by Reinberg, A., Vieux, N. and Andlauer, P., pp. 263–270, Oxford, Pergamon Press.

Farrell, D. and Stamm, C.L. (1988) Meta-analysis of the correlates of employee absence. *Hum. Relations*, **41**, 211–227.

Fischer, F.M. (1986) Retrospective study regarding absenteeism among shiftworkers. *Int. Arch. Occup. Environ. Health*, **58**, 301–320.

Folkard, S. and Monk, T.H. (1979) Shiftwork and performance. *Hum. Factors*, **21**, 483–492.

Folkard, S., Monk, T.H. and Lobban, M.C. (1978) Short and long-term adjustment of circadian rhythms in 'permanent' night nurses. *Ergonomics*, **21**, 785–799.

Hamelin, P. (1987) Lorry drivers' time habits in work and their involvement in traffic accidents. *Ergonomics*, **30**, 1323–1333.

Hildebrandt, G., Rohmert, W. and Rutenfranz, J. (1974) Twelve and 24 hour rhythms in error frequency of locomotive drivers and the influence of tiredness. *Int. J. Chronobiol.*, **2**, 175–180.

Khaleque, A. and Verhaegen, P. (1981) Circadian effects in short-cycle repetitive work in a two-shift system. In *Night and Shift Work: Biological and Social Aspects*, edited by Reinberg, A., Vieux, N. and Andlauer, pp. 409–416, Oxford: Pergamon.

Lauber, J.K. and Kayten, P.J. (1988) Keynote Address: Sleepiness, circadian dysrhythmia, and fatigue in transportation system accidents. *Sleep*, **11**, 503–512.

Meers, A. (1975) Performance on different turns of duty within a three-shift system and its relation to body temperature – Two field studies. In *Experimental Studies of Shiftwork*, edited by Colquhoun, P., Folkard, S., Knauth, P. and Rutenfranz, J., pp. 188–205, Opladen: Westdeutscher Verlag.

Monk, T.H. and Embrey, D.E. (1981) A field study of circadian rhythms in actual and interpolated task performance. In *Night and Shift Work: Biological and Social Aspects*, edited by Reinberg, A., Vieux, N. and Andlauer, P., pp. 473–480, Oxford: Pergamon Press.

Monk, T.H. and Folkard, S. (1985) Shiftwork and performance. In *Hours of Work – Temporal Factors in Work Scheduling*, edited by Folkard, S. and Monk, T.H., pp. 239–252, New York: John Wiley & Sons.

Moog, R. (1987) Optimization of shift work: Physiological contributions, *Ergonomics*, **30**, 1249–1259.

Prokop, O. and Prokop, L. (1955) Ermunudung und Einschlafen am Steuer, Zentralblatt fur Verkehrs-Medizin. *Verkehrs-Psychologie und angrenzende Gebiete*, **1**, 19–30.

Tepas, D.I., Walsh, J.K. and Armstrong, D.R. (1981a) Comprehensive study of the sleep of shift workers. In *The Twenty-four Hour Workday: Proceedings of a Symposium on Variations in Work–Sleep Schedules*, edited by Johnson, L.C., Tepas, D.I., Colquhoun, W.P. and Colligan, M.J., pp. 419–433, Cincinnati, OH: Department of Health and Human Services (NIOSH).

Tepas, D.I., Walsh, J.K., Moss, P.D. and Armstrong, D.R. (1981b), Polysomnographic correlates of shiftworker performance in the laboratory. In *Night and Shift Work: Biological and Social Aspects*, edited by Reinberg, A., Vieux, N. and Andlauer, P., pp. 179–186, Oxford: Pergamon Press.

Tilley, A.J., Wilkinson, R.T., Warren, P.S.G., Watson, B. and Drud, M. (1982) The sleep and performance of shift workers. *Hum. Factors*, **24**, 629–641.

Wojtczak-Jaroszowa, J. and Pawlowska-Skyba, K. (1967) Night and shift work. I: Circadian variations in work. *Med. Pr.*, **18**, 1.

Wojtczak-Jaroszowa, J. and Jarosz, D. (1987) Chronohygienic and chronosocial aspects of industrial accidents. *Prog. Clin. Biol. Res.*, **227B**, 415–426.

Wojtczak-Jaroszowa, J., Makowska, Z., Rzepechi, A., Banaszkiewicz, A. and Romejko, A. (1978) Changes in psychomotor and mental task performance following physical work in standard conditions, and in a shift-working situation. *Ergonomics*, **21**, 801–809.

Chapter 7

Inter-individual differences

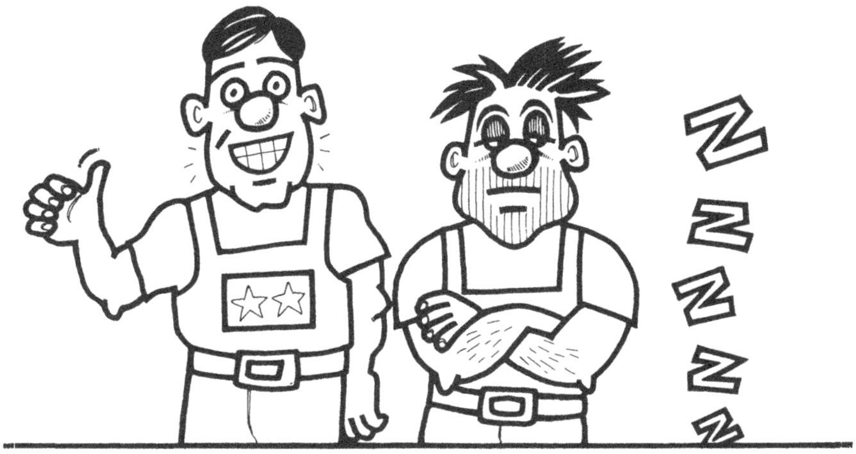

Introduction

As even the most cursory of observations will confirm, any group of shift workers can be divided into three groups: those coping reasonably well, those who have some problems but are 'getting by', and those who are having serious problems and are barely able to cope. This chapter discusses whether it is possible *a priori* to determine who is likely to fall into these groups.

Age and experience

Although old age does not always bring wisdom, it invariably brings experience. Most 50-year-old shift workers have had several decades of experience in coping with the abnormal routines that shift work requires, and developing the strategies and techniques needed to cope with them. Moreover, housing conditions for such workers have often improved with seniority and sleeping conditions quietened as children have grown up and left home. From these improvements, and from the conventional wisdom that 50 year olds need less sleep than 20 year olds, it could be predicted that shift work coping ability would improve with age and experience. Unfortunately, the reverse is true. Both age and experience are negative factors regarding shift work coping ability (Foret *et al.*, 1981).

The sleep of the late middle-aged and elderly is different from that of the young (Miles and Dement, 1980). It can be characterized as being more 'fragile', i.e. shorter, more easily disrupted, more fragmented and lighter. Interestingly, exactly the same characterization can be used to describe the day sleep of night workers (Akerstedt, 1985). It appears that older people may be less able to achieve as much sleep as the young rather than simply needing less. Negative effects of age and day sleeps may well be additive, precipitating a major sleep disorder for the individual concerned. Differences between old and young also exist in variables related to the circadian system. Advancing age is characterized by low amplitude, early phased circadian rhythms (Weitzman *et al.*, 1982), perhaps due to a shortening of the 'natural' period of the endogenous circadian pacemaker (Monk, 1989). Such a change is associated with a move towards 'morningness', i.e. earlier bedtimes and waketimes (with the direction of causality unclear) (Monk *et al.*, 1991). Unfortunately, as we discuss later, the characteristic of 'circadian type' (of which morningness is but one measure) is for all age groups one of the best predictors of those who are likely to have shift work coping problems (Monk and Folkard, 1985). Thus the 'morningness' consequence of ageing can itself render shift work adjustment difficult. Also important is the issue of phase lability – i.e. the rate at which the circadian system can re-align to be appropriate to a new routine. Although direct laboratory comparisons have only just been made, indirect cross-study comparisons suggest that the circadian rhythms of middle-aged people are slower to re-align (phase shift) to an acute change in routine than are those of the young (Moline *et al.*, 1991). The picture is, however, confused, since Reinberg has blamed age-related shift work intolerance (to the rapid rotation schedules typical in France) on increased phase lability (i.e. faster re-alignment) consequent upon reduced amplitudes (Reinberg *et al.*, 1980). A possible explanation comes from his more recent work which showed a complete loss of 24-hour entrainment in elderly intolerant shift workers (i.e. a breakdown in the circadian entrainment system altogether) leading to low amplitude 24-hour rhythms (Reinberg *et al.*, 1984).

In another French study, Foret (Foret *et al.*, 1981) addressed the question of whether experience with shift work was a positive or negative factor regarding sleep disorders. Considering age and experience separately, he showed convincingly that both were negative factors, a finding confirmed by Czeisler in an unpublished US study. An Austrian shift worker survey by Koller (Koller *et al.*, 1978) revealed that fewer than 20% expected to continue shift work right up until retirement.

With increasing trends towards the elimination of age discrimination, and grass-roots pressure for jobs in the older age group, problems of age-related intolerance to shift work may become a significant crisis. Pressure will be particularly great in the late 1990s when most of the baby-boom generation enter their fifties. It could well be that the turn of the century sees a plethora of new shift working positions with insufficient people willing or able to fill them.

Personality and circadian type

There are three broad classifications of human 'circadian type'. The first and most popular relates to the phase or timing of preferred behaviour. It is a widely-held belief that the human population can be divided into 'morning larks' and 'night owls'. 'Morning larks' (M-types) are characterized as being 'early to bed and early to rise', up and about at the crack of dawn, but fading fast by mid-evening. In contrast, evening active 'night owls' (E-types) are at their best well into the late evening, but have much more trouble waking up in the morning. Attempts to quantify this aspect of human inter-individual difference started in Sweden in the late 1960s with the work of Oquist and Patkai (1971) who developed pencil-and-paper questionnaires of morningness, and showed scores on them to relate (at the extremes) to time-of-day differences in various physiological and psychological measures. The best known English language morningness test was developed by Horne and Ostberg (1976), building upon that work, and testing the questionnaire on a group of British undergraduates. Although other (and, perhaps, better) English language morningness tests have been developed (Torsvall and Akerstedt, 1980; Smith *et al.*, 1989), none has achieved the widespread acceptance enjoyed by the Horne-Ostberg instrument. More than 50 recent publications have cited the work; studies have used it to divide subjects into M-types and E-types (often as extremes) and shown different time of day effects in various physiological and psychological measures.

There are three reasons why M-types have more difficulty with shift work than E-types. First is the prosaic one that M-types find it hard to stay awake at night and to sleep in late during the morning hours, precisely the behaviour required of a night worker. Secondly, there is the fact that E-types may be that way because they are less susceptible than M-types to the surrounding physical and social time cues (zeitgebers). Because the human circadian rhythms naturally tends to 'free-run' slowly (typically to about a 25 hour day) such effects would naturally lead to E-type behaviour. Thirdly, there is the likelihood that morningness is related to that 'free-running' period length, with M-types having a length of 24.3 hours, for example, and E-types on 25.5 hours. Because night work usually requires a phase delay in behaviour (e.g. a 9.00 am bedtime, rather than a midnight one) a long free-running period would be of obvious benefit.

There are a number of different ways in which one can become an E-type as opposed to an M-type, and it is thus uncertain whether morningness is truly a trait variable. In particular, a longer than average 'free-running' or natural circadian period (e.g. 25.4 hours), a weaker entrainment mechanism (i.e. a less effective process of resetting the timing of the circadian system), or a weaker (more chaotic) set of time cues (zeitgebers) will all tend to create an E-type rather than an M-type. Moreover, several factor analyses of Horne-Ostberg scores have suggested that the scale may not be truly unidimensional, suggesting the value of additional multifaceted circadian type scales.

In the 1970s, we worked on the development of a second approach, namely a Circadian Type questionnaire (CTQ) designed to evaluate three circadian factors: morningness (CTQ-M), sleep pattern rigidity (CTQ-Rs) and vigour (CTQ-V) (Folkard *et al.*, 1979). The CTQ-M scale is broadly analogous to Horne and Ostberg's morningness scale. The Rs scale relates to the trait of keeping to the same bedtime and waketime, irrespective of the needs of the situation. The high CTQ-Rs individuals tend to keep to the same bedtimes even on vacation, and find it difficult to sleep at unusual times of the day. The CTQ-V scale related to vigour as compared with languor, high CTQ-V types are 'hale and hearty'. The CTQ has now been used in several different laboratories, is cited in more than 25 recent publications, and has been translated into German, Polish, Italian and Serbo-Croatian. Generally speaking, those scoring high on CTQ-V and low on CTQ-R, have been found to suffer less as a result of shift work.

A third approach to quantifying inter-individual circadian differences comes from consideration of personality factors, in particular those of neuroticism and extraversion. Using the Heron Personality Inventory, Blake (1967) showed that neurotic extroverts had later peaking circadian temperature rhythms than neurotic introverts. Using both the Heron and the more popular Eysenck Personality Inventory (Eysenck and Eysenck, 1963) neurotic introverts were also shown to be less able than neurotic extroverts to cope with shift work, jet-lag (Colquhoun and Folkard, 1978) and daylight saving time changes (Monk and Aplin, 1980).

Habitual sleep need

In addition to the above-mentioned characteristics, the simple one of habitual sleep need can be a potent predictor, particularly at the extremes (Box 7.1). Those who habitually need 9 hours or more of sleep to feel refreshed invariably find shift work almost impossible to cope with, while those needing 5 hours or less invariably find it easy. This effect suggests one biological reason why women may find shift work more difficult to cope with than men. In a study of sleep fractions (% time asleep) performed by Wever (1979) from a number of free-running studies, women were found to need about 90 minutes more sleep per 24 hour day than men. Probably much more important as a gender difference, however, is the societal one, whereby extensive home making and child care roles are expected of women, in addition to their shift work burden (Chapter 3).

Box 7.1

A 33-three year-old married security officer, Wife works part-time, two children at school. Irregular shift system.

> I work with people who seem to be able to cope with less sleep than me but my own personal feeling is if I can't get eight hours sleep then I don't feel sufficiently rested, if you understand what I mean. I can tell if I've missed an hour or two sleep and I feel as though I need to catch it up at some time, either by going to bed earlier the following day or having a lie-in the following morning.

Shift worker selection

The points raised in this chapter, together with the health issues discussed in Chapter 5, give rise to the beginnings of a classification of those who could be at added risk for shift work coping problems of one sort or another. Tepas and Monk (1987) have collected them into a table (Table 9.1), and although some of the precise ordering may be debatable, the overall impression holds true.

Having reproduced this table, it is important to realize, however, that such information should only be used as a counselling guide, rather than as precise selection criteria. There are many people in the high risk categories who are coping very well with shift work. Present knowledge does not permit an accurate classification of precisely who will and who will not cope well with shift work. It is thus premature to exclude people from shift work simply because their classification appears in Table 9.1 or because they happen to score high on a scale of morningness, for example.

Table 9.1 Factors within an individual that are likely to cause shift work coping problems

Over 50 years of age
Second job for pay ('moonlighting')
Heavy domestic work load
'Morning type' individuals ('larks')
History of sleep disorders
Neurotic introvert
Psychiatric illness
History of alcohol or drug abuse
History of gastrointestinal complaints
Epilepsy
Diabetes
Heart disease

Conclusions

Some people cope quite well with shift work, others rather badly. Those coping badly are often in late middle-age, morning-types, rigid pattern and/or long sleeper categories. However, although our knowledge may permit some counselling regarding shift work suitability, it is probably insufficiently refined to permit actual employee selection.

References

Akerstedt, T. (1985) Adjustment of physiological circadian rhythms and the sleep-wake cycle to shiftwork. In *Hours of Work: Temporal Factors in Work Scheduling*, edited by Folkard, S. and Monk, T.H., pp. 185–197, New York: John Wiley & Sons.

Blake, M.J.F. (1967) Relationship between circadian rhythm of body temperature and introversion–extraversion. *Nature*, **215**, 896–897.

Colquhoun, W.P. and Folkard, S. (1978) Personality differences in body-temperature rhythm, and their relation to its adjustment to night work. *Ergonomics*, **21**, 811–817.

Eysenck, H.J. and Eysenck, S.B. (1963) *Eysenck Personality Inventory*, London: University of London Press.

Folkard, S., Monk, T.H. and Lobban, M.C. (1979) Towards a predictive test of adjustment to shiftwork. *Ergonomics*, **22**, 79–91.

Foret, J., Bensimon, G., Benoit, O. and Vieux, N. (1981) Quality of sleep as a function of age and shift work. In *Night and Shift Work: Biological and Social Aspects*, edited by Reinberg, A., Vieux, N. and Andlauer, P., pp. 149–160, Oxford: Pergamon Press.

Horne, J.A. and Ostberg, O. (1976) A self-assessment questionnaire to determine morningness–eveningness in human circadian rhythms. *Int. J. Chronobiol.*, **4**, 97–110.

Koller, M., Kundi, M. and Cervinka, R. (1978) Field studies of shiftwork at an Austrian oil refinery. I: Health and psychosocial well-being of workers who drop out of shiftwork. *Ergonomics*, **21**, 835–847.

Miles, L. and Dement, W.C. (1980) Sleep and aging. *Sleep*, **3**, 119–220.

Moline, M.L., Pollak, C.P., Monk, T.H. *et al.* (1991) Age-related differences in recovery from simulated jet lag. *Sleep*, **14**(5), 42–48.

Monk, T.H. (1989) Sleep disorders in the elderly. *Clin. Ger. Med.*, **5**, 331–346.

Monk, T.H. and Aplin, L.C. (1980) Spring and autumn daylight saving time changes: Studies of adjustment in sleep timings, mood, and efficiency. *Ergonomics*, **23**, 167–178.

Monk, T.H. and Folkard, S. (1985) Individual differences in shiftwork adjustment. In *Hours of Work – Temporal Factors in Work Scheduling*, edited by Folkard, S. and Monk, T.H., pp. 227–237, New York: John Wiley & Sons.

Monk, T.H., Reynolds, C.F., Buysse, D.J. *et al.* (1991) Circadian characteristics of healthy 80 year olds and their relationship to objectively recorded sleep. *J. Gerontol. (Med. Sci.)*, **46**, M171–175.

Patkai, P. (1971) Interindividual differences in diurnal variations in alertness, performance, and adrenaline excretion. *Acta Physiol. Scand.*, **81**, 35–46.

Reinberg, A., Andlauer, P., Guillet, P., Nicolai, A., Vieux, N. and Laporte, A. (1980) Oral temperature, circadian rhythm amplitude, ageing and tolerance to shiftwork. *Ergonomics*, **23**, 55–64.

Reinberg, A., Andlauer, P., DePrins, J., Malbecq, W., Vieux, N. and Bourdeleau, P. (1984) Desynchronization of the oral temperature circadian rhythm and intolerance to shift work. *Nature*, **308**, 272–274.

Smith, C.S., Reilly, C. and Midkiff, K. (1989) Evaluations of three circadian rhythm questionnaires with suggestions for an improved measure of morningness. *J. Appl. Psychol.*, **74**, 728–738.
Tepas, D.I. and Monk, T.H. (1987) Work schedules. In *Handbook of Human Factors*, edited by Salvendy, G., pp. 819–843, New York: John Wiley & Sons.
Torsvall, L. and Akerstedt, T. (1980) A diurnal type scale: Construction, consistency, and validation in shift work. *Scand. J. Work. Environ. Health*, **6**, 283–290.
Weitzman, E.D., Moline, M.L., Czeisler, C.A. and Zimmerman, J.C. (1982) Chronobiology of aging: Temperature, sleep–wake rhythms and entrainment. *Neurobiol. Aging*, **3**, 299–309.
Wever, R.A. (1979) *The Circadian System of Man: Results of Experiments Under Temporal Isolation*, New York: Springer-Verlag.

Chapter 8

Coping strategies for the worker

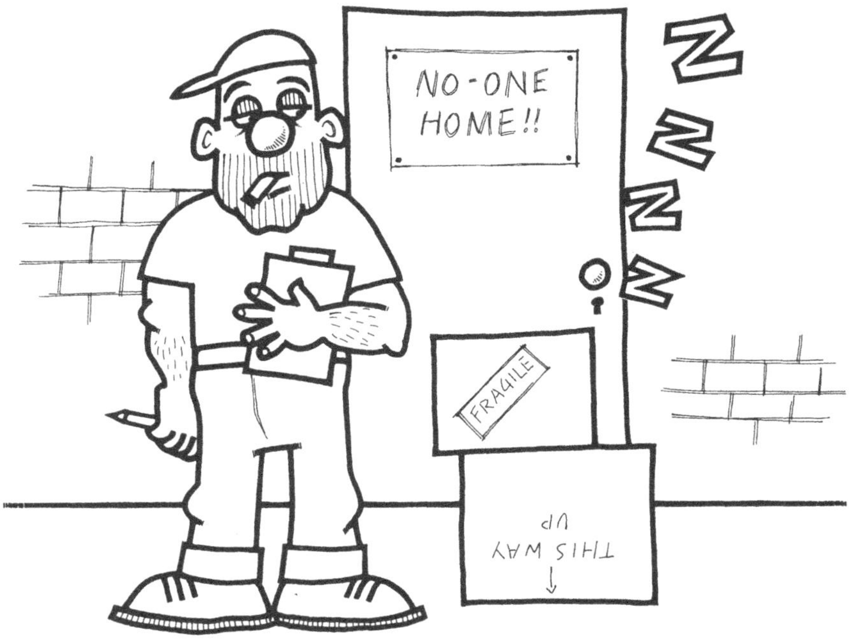

Sleep, circadian and domestic solutions

Introduction

As we have seen in previous chapters, shift work is a multifaceted problem that therefore requires multifaceted solutions. There are two major criticisms that can be levelled at the shift work research community. The first is that we tend to concentrate much more on describing and cataloguing all the problems of shift work, rather than addressing ourselves to possible solutions to those problems, and secondly, that when we do put forward a solution it is usually a single solution in one particular domain. Thus, for example, shift work research experts have put forward solutions based on feasting and fasting diets (Ehret, 1981), changes in the direction and speed of shift rotation (Czeisler *et al.*, 1982), exercise regimens (Ilmarinen *et al.*, 1980) and bright lights (Czeisler *et al.*, 1990); concentrating on those solutions to the exclusion of other facets of the shift work problem which may be equally important. There is no one single solution to shift work; there is no one coping strategy that the shift worker can adopt to ameliorate his or her problem at a stroke. Instead, solutions to the shift work problem must proceed along a number of different fronts. In previous chapters we have categorized the strain inherent in shift work according to three different areas: sleep, the circadian system, and the social and domestic situation. Any solution that will help the shift worker to cope with shift work must address all three areas of this triad.

Sleep strategies

The goal that the shift worker seeks to achieve in relation to sleep is simple: trying to get enough of it. Almost every survey of shift worker problems comes up with sleep as a major factor (Knauth *et al*., 1980). Despite this, most shift workers consciously or unconsciously 'cheat' on their sleep, not giving it the attention it deserves. It is vitally important for shift workers to realize that sleep is as important to them as oxygen and that they should treat it that way. They must not let social or domestic pressures eat into their sleep time.

Figure 8.1 illustrates the results of two surveys, one from Germany the other from Japan, each involving more than 2000 respondents (Kogi, 1985), plotting the number of hours of sleep obtained as a function of the time of day it is started. The startling reduction in sleep duration during daylight hours is a function of both voluntary and involuntary (circadian) processes.

Shift workers should realize that if they find themselves spending most of their 'weekend' break catching up on sleep, they have not been getting enough sleep during the week and are heading for significant shift work coping problems. The loss of off-duty time to sleep can create additional problems both in the circadian and the social and domestic arena; shift workers should therefore strive to preserve sleep opportunities during the working week.

Unless an individual is sick or chronically sleep deprived, it is not possible to have a span of refreshing sleep totally at will; both the body and the mind have to be made ready for sleep. Regularity of sleep

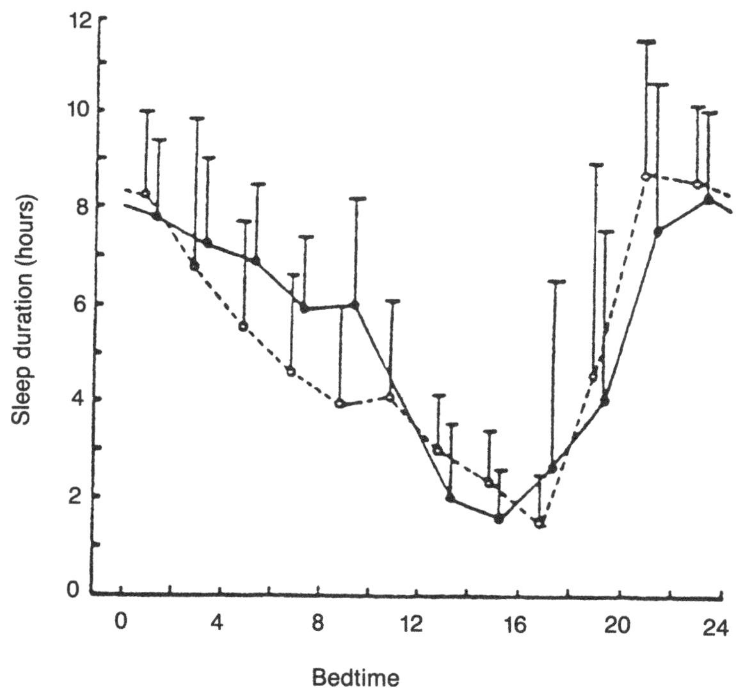

Figure 8.1 Mean and standard deviation of sleep length of German (N = 2332) and Japanese (N = 3240) shift workers in studies summarized by Kogi (1985).

patterns is a vitally important component of coping behaviour and is of course directly related to the circadian rhythms discussed in Chapter 2 and in the following section. A simple rule that shift workers should take to heart is that a correctly set biological clock is the single most important factor in ensuring good sleep and fewer jet-lag type effects. To the extent made possible by their work and domestic routines, shift workers should be highly regular in their sleeping patterns and should consciously avoid a 'snacking' approach to sleep, whereby they grab it wherever and whenever they can. The process of taking naps should only be regarded as an emergency catching-up process, coping with acute sleep decrements as they occur, rather than as an integral part of the shift worker's overall general sleep strategy. The only exception to this might be an afternoon or evening nap before the first night shift of a run of night duty.

As part of the general cavalier attitude towards sleep that many shift workers exhibit, there is often a tendency to take sleep on the couch in front of the TV or in otherwise unsatisfacotry sleep environments. This is wrong; the shift worker should have as regular and as an elaborate bedtime ritual as the day worker. He or she should set the stage for their sleep: darkening a bedroom with heavy curtains and going through all of the teeth cleaning, bathroom use and nightwear rituals that are usual for an ordinary night's sleep. The adoption of such rituals not only serves as a stimulus to the shift worker, preparing him or her for sleep, but also reinforces to the family around the shift worker the point that this sleep is as important to the shift worker's life as the night sleep of day working members of the household. A sign on the door reading 'shift worker asleep' may emphasize the importance of protecting the sleep of the shift worker. As part of that emphasis the telephone ringer should be switched off, the doorbell disconnected, and family members instructed to preserve this time as one of quiet and sleep availability for the shift worker. Other social aspects are discussed in a later section.

Sleep clinicians have developed patterns of behaviour described as 'sleep hygiene' (Hauri, 1983). Sleep hygiene consists of a set of rules and procedures which can often be very helpful to people suffering from insomnia. Some of them we have discussed already, such as teeth cleaning, bathroom use and nightwear rituals, and regularity of sleeping habits. Other aspects relate to consideration of the stimulus that the bedroom setting supplies to the individual concerned (Dorsey, 1991). For some people the bedroom can become a situation associated with stress and unpleasantness. At the extreme this is exemplified by the insomniac who dreads going into a bedroom because he or she 'knows' that a night of frustration and tossing and turning awaits them. The aim of sleep hygiene, as it relates to stimulus control, is to ensure that the bedroom is only associated in the mind of the sleeper with pleasant and relaxing experiences. To accomplish this, it is vital that the bedroom only be used for sleep and lovemaking. Paying bills, watching TV and discussing family problems should all take place in other rooms of the house. They should not take place in bed. If an individual finds that they cannot sleep and starts to become tense and frustrated then they should leave the bedroom, read for 20 minutes in a different room, and then go back to bed so that the frustration occurs in a different room. The shift worker has two things working against them: they are in a stressful situation and they very often have a biological clock which is not preparing them satisfactorily for a long bout of sleep. If there are additional stresses that come from poor sleep hygiene, this will simply compound the problem, resulting in a significant loss of sleep for the person concerned.

Part of sleep hygiene also relates to the consumption of 'uppers' and 'downers'. Sleeping pills will be discussed in a later section of this chapter. More frequently used by shift workers are caffeine and alcohol. It is important for the shift worker to remember that caffeine stays in the bloodstream for at least five hours (Buysse, 1991). Shift workers should not drink any caffeinated drink (and that includes tea and caffeinated soft drinks) within five hours of their expected bedtime. They should also avoid the trap of using alcohol to help 'put themselves to sleep'; for most night workers getting to sleep is not the problem, staying asleep and getting the right sort of sleep and depth of sleep is the problem, and unfortunately alcohol is likely to make that a lot more difficult (Yules, 1966).

Eating lightly before bedtime and avoiding caffeine and alcohol is likely to increase the continuity and depth of the sleep that the shift worker obtains. Some people find a warm milk drink helpful in this, although the scientific evidence for such beneficial effects has yet to be determined. Others will use different techniques to help them. Overall, the aim should be (1) to preserve a regular fixed interval of time that is solely dedicated to sleep; and (2) to adopt behaviour patterns and rituals that both reinforce the sanctity of that sleeping interval, and which help the individual to associate the sleeping episode with pleasant and relaxing feelings.

Circadian system

As we have discussed in earlier chapters there is a biological clock or circadian system inside the head which has a momentum of its own and which is resistant to abrupt changes in routine. The purpose of that clock is to prepare the body and brain for sleep at certain times of the day and active wakefulness at others. The biological clock lowers body temperature, heart rate and blood pressure, suppresses the excretion of hormones such as cortisol which result in wakefulness, and increases the excretion of hormones such as melatonin which help the individual to feel drowsy (Arendt *et al.*, 1989). The biological clock also protects the sleep by suppressing renal and bowel functions and hunger so that an acceptably long bout of sleep can be obtained.

As Professor Jim Horne (1988) has pointed out in his recent book, it is not natural for human beings to go for 7 or 8 hours without using the toilet, without having something to eat or drink, and without moving about. It is a time of fasting and it is a time of energy depletion. If, as an organism, we are to cope with this interval of fasting, tissue depletion and energy depletion, then certain functions must be depressed by the biological clock. That means that if the biological clock has not done its job for any reason, a number of different symptoms will arise in the shift worker. The shift worker's digestion may be affected, he or she may need to use the toilet during their day sleep episode, and/or might find a muddled-headedness and irritability while awake. All of these symptoms come from the one basic problem that the circadian system is not correctly aligned with the routine that the shift worker is trying to live (Monk, 1988) (Box 8.1).

The biological clock or circadian system has no magical way of telling which is night and which is day. At present there is no known

Box 8.1

From a 34-year-old married male security officer. Wife works part-time, two children at school. Irregular shift schedule.

> I've worked shifts ever since I've known my wife. I've worked shifts right from when we've been married and we've been married 11 years. So my wife has never known me work anything other than shifts and she still, although she's lived with me for all of these years, she still cannot understand why I feel tired after I've been in bed for eight hours after a night shift. But to me it's not the same sort of quality of sleep, it's not like a deep sleep. You never seem to get into that deep restful sleep. It's more of a cat nap sleep right the way through the day if you like. Plus you get woken up by the daytime noises. I come home from work at about 5.30–5.45 am, get washed and changed and I'm in bed by 6 o'clock. I like to get into bed as soon as I can so that I can get off to sleep before the sun comes up and before the children get up to go to school, etc. I get off to sleep quite easy to begin with, but that seems to be my best sleep period at the beginning, and as the day wears on the quality of sleep gets worse and worse and I seem to get to the point that, however much I lie there and will myself to get to sleep, I just can't.
>
> Very often daytime noises wake me up, like the dustbin men come round or the children might be outside playing [etc.]. But I also wake up by myself, without anything waking me up, and I think 'Oh what time is it' and look across and it might be 9, 10 or 11 o'clock. It's usually around that period that I wake up. Now usually when I wake up I think I'll go to the toilet, so I go to the toilet. Well once I've staggered out of the bedroom into the daylight of the bathroom, after a minute or so your eyes become accustomed to the daylight and you think 'I might as well stop up and have a cup of tea now.' You don't feel tired enough to go back to bed. But by that time you feel fairly refreshed. So what I'll do is I'll make myself a cup of tea and I might have a read of the paper or watch TV for an hour, by which time I feel very often as though I could get back to sleep again so I go back to bed get myself comfortable and very often I can get back to sleep again. So it's like a disturbed sleep cycle if you like. Now if I work a longer time, let's say I work a night shift cycle which lasts more than three or four night shifts, my body seems to become more accustomed to that night shift cycle and the longer I'm on it the more rested I feel. That broken sleep period in the day seems to disappear and it is possible for me to sleep through to 3 or 4 in the afternoon.

chronobiotic or pill which can be taken reliably to reset the circadian system. Thus, we cannot directly affect the circadian system itself. All the system can go on is the information it is given. In developing suitable sleep/wake patterns this flow of information into the circadian system must be manipulated in order to improve the chances of obtaining the desired effect. We do this using time cues or zeitgebers. Zeitgebers are the time cues that impinge on the individual and, by doing so, allow the circadian system to distinguish between night and day and to run at the correct period length (Wever, 1979).

In moving towards a solution, the shift worker has to consider which time cues are going to work in favour of shift work adjustment and which are going to work against it. Clearly, before that decision can be made it must be known just where in time the biological clock is to be pointed, that is, at which times sleep and wakefulness are expected.

It will also be necessary to know which time cues are strong and which are comparatively weak. Here there is some debate in the literature. Throughout the 1970s, most experts agreed that the cycle of daylight and darkness was not a very important zeitgeber for human beings (Wever, 1979). In 1980 however, the attention focused on a hormone in the blood called melatonin. This hormone makes people feel sleepy when circulating in the bloodstream and seems to be an important part of the biological clock. Peak levels of melatonin in the bloodstream usually occur at night, but Professor Lewy and colleagues (1980) found that they could eliminate that peak by putting the individual in extremely bright levels of illumination at night. Such levels approximated those we experience in daylight, but not the levels that normal room lighting give (Lewy *et al*., 1980). Further work along these lines determined that daylight illumination levels have a special role in human beings as time cues, being particularly strong as resetters of the biological clock (Wever *et al*., 1983; Czeisler *et al*., 1986). This is in contrast to lower animals, in whom entrainment can be achieved by extremely low levels of illumination. There has since been research on using bright levels of illumination to help shift workers to reset their biological clocks. This will be discussed in a later section.

As well as daylight and darkness it is clear that there are many other factors and effects that can act as time cues for the human being. Patterns of eating and sleeping, social interaction, noise and temperature levels have all been shown to be important zeitgebers for the human. Patterns of activity in particular have been shown to act as internal zeitgebers reinforcing the need for regularity in an individual's sleep/wake cycling strategy.

The particular circadian strategy that the shift worker should adopt will depend upon the type of shift schedule he or she is required to work. The first classification relates to the speed of shift rotation. Shift rotas are discussed in greater detail in Chapter 9. Essentially, a distinction can be made between rapid, intermediate and slow rotation. In rapid shift rotation all shift timings are worked within a given week. A typical example of this is the metropolitan rota comprising of two morning shifts, two afternoon shifts, two night shifts and two days off. Intermediate shift rotations are the weekly rotating schedules, where a week at one shift timing is followed by a week at a different shift timing. The long shift rotations comprise 2, 3 or 4 weeks at a particular shift timing before the individual changes to a different timing.

For the rapid rotation the circadian aim is very simple. The shift worker should seek to retain a day orientation, that is a diurnal routine. He or she should try to be as much like a day worker in their zeitgeber exposure as possible. Thus, they should seek to experience daylight levels of illumination during the day, they should avoid a heavy night shift 'lunchtime' meal, and should even consider taking a quick nap during their lunch break part way through the night shift. All of these activities will, of course, lead to feelings of sleepiness during the night shift, and the shift worker should aggressively adopt some of the strategies related to maintaining nighttime alertness that are discussed later in this chapter.

For the intermediate and long rotation speeds the issue is more complicated. Basically, the first aim should be rapidly to acquire and maintain a circadian orientation which is appropriate to the particular shift timing that is being worked. We will concentrate on night work, because that is the shift timing that is associated with the greatest circadian changes. Typically, the aim will be to reset the circadian system so that it expects work from, say, midnight to 8 am and sleep from 9 am to 4 pm. Note first that this is not simply a mirror image inversion but a delay of about 9 hours. Instead of going to bed at midnight the shift worker is retiring at 9 am, and waking up (ideally) about 7 hours later at 4 pm. The distinction between a delay and inversion is important because the biological clock copes more easily with delays than with advances in routine (see Chapter 2). Adjustment to a 6-hour phase advance, for example, can take just as long as that to a 9-hour delay (Aschoff *et al.*, 1975). The first major recommendation to the night worker is therefore to go to bed as soon as possible after the end of the night shift. He or she should get home, have a light meal, perhaps a warm milk drink, and go to bed. Invariably shift workers find that the earlier they get to bed after a night shift the more sleep they will obtain (see Figure 8.1). This is because the earlier they go to bed the smaller the amount of adjustment their biological clock has to make. The number of interruptions in sleep that they experience, and the amount of 'jet-lag' they feel will also be reduced. It is important to avoid the temptation to do domestic chores or watch TV first. This will unnecessarily delay the onset of sleep, and will inevitably make matters worse rather than better.

Naps should only be used as a 'topping-up' process before going to work on the night shift. A major sleep episode in the evening is, anyway, usually very difficult to obtain because temperature is then approaching its peak. Secondly, it represents a phase advance rather than a phase delay in routine. This is harder for the circadian system to accomplish and we should remember that the timing of sleep can itself act as a zeitgeber. Regularity of sleep is important in teaching the biological clock where it should be putting sleep, and where wakefulness.

Sleep is not the only time cue to which the biological clock will pay attention, however. As mentioned earlier, daylight levels of illumination may be an extremely strong time cue for the human circadian system. Unless the workplace has the availability of daylight illumination levels at night through the provision of special lighting (see next chapter), it may be important for the shift worker to avoid daylight illumination levels on his or her drive home from work. It might, therefore, be helpful for shift workers to wear dark sunglasses on their way home from work, especially if they live to the east of their place of work and find themselves driving into the sunrise. This makes sense from a hormonal point of view. As we mentioned before, melatonin is only suppressed by daylight levels of illumination, and avoiding melatonin suppression during the journey home may assist in the phase adjustment process of the biological clock. With respect to the evening, Dr Charmane Eastman (1987) and her colleagues of Chicago are performing studies aimed at determining whether a bank of really bright artificial lights may be helpful in the late evening prior to coming on shift. It is, as yet too early to definitely say whether such countermeasures are worth the time and expense involved, but there is some evidence that they might be helpful. Probably more useful would be daylight levels of illumination at the actual workplace. This is discussed in greater detail in the following chapter concerned with employer interventions.

Other time cues that the shift worker's circadian system will pay attention to are meal times and other aspects of the daily routine. The more regular that routine is, the more powerful it will be in helping the circadian system to be appropriately aligned to the work routine. The shift worker should try and take a regular three meals a day and to try to keep them at predictable times as much as possible, given the work schedule. Large organizations such as hospitals, which have good canteen facilities for their night shift workers, can find a significant improvement in shift work coping ability compared with those without such facilities. This improvement will also relate to some of the gastro-intestinal problems that have been discussed in Chapter 5. In summary, everything the shift worker can do to regularize his or her routine will help the biological clock to adjust.

The complication in intermediate and slow shift rotation speed, concerns what happens as the shift worker reaches the 'weekend' break. At the beginning of that break they have a couple of days off in front of them. The question then is: what should they do now? Should they attempt to keep the nocturnal circadian orientation or should they revert to a normal diurnal routine? The answer to that question depends on whether they will be moving to a morning or evening shift after the break, or whether they will be remaining on the night shift because the shift system is a very slowly rotating or fixed one. If the shift worker is going to be changing to a morning or evening shift after the break then he or she will be aiming to reset their biological clock towards a diurnal orientation, that is towards sleep at night. It is therefore best for such shift workers to have short (2 hours or less) sleep after coming off the last night shift of the week and then allow themselves a good long night's sleep during the days off (Box 8.2). Such night sleeps will be helped by the fact that the day sleep preceding them is of a short duration. This, of course, makes sense from a social and domestic point of view too, especially if there are children who have to be taken to scout meetings, soccer games, etc.

The circadian advantage that such shift workers will have is that all of the powerful time cues (zeitgebers) which were working against the shift worker on the night shift are now working in their favour in rapidly re-establishing the day active orientation of the biological clock. In studies of circadian rhythms following such 'weekend' breaks it has been found that reversion to a diurnal routine can be extremely rapid (Van Loon, 1963; Monk, 1986). The process of acquiring a nocturnal orientation can be likened to that of a salmon leaping up a waterfall, where the top of the waterfall represents a nocturnal orientation and the bottom a diurnal one. It is extremely hard to make it up to that nocturnal orientation but all too easy, because of the powerful zeitgebers involved, to revert down to the diurnal orientation.

A very different approach has to be taken if the shift worker is on a permanent night system, or is on a slowly rotating nights on system.

> **Box 8.2**
>
> From a 46-year-old male print room supervisor. Wife part-time teacher, two teenage children. Rotating shifts, 90 nights a year.
>
> > On the last morning after a run of six nights, before four days off, I finish at 8 am and go to bed for 2 hours perhaps, not more than three. If someone is around the house I ask them to wake me at about 11 and I'll sort of hang around the house all day and go to bed at 11 in the evening. Even though I go to bed at 11, I still do not sleep until 1–2 am, but once I get to sleep I sleep for about 6 hours. I get up the next day and the night shift is out of my system.

Here the aim should be to retain as much of the circadian system's night active orientation as possible. Thus, the aim is to stay nocturnal, and for certain individuals and certain isolated situations that can easily be accomplished. However, for most people, who have children, commitments and outside relationships, it is usually extremely difficult (Box 8.3). Compromises can and should be made. The shift worker should get up as late as they can in the morning given their commitments and then go to bed correspondingly later in the night; they should wear dark sunglasses or stay indoors during the morning hours, trying to stick to their old meal schedule as much as they can. It is not easy of course, shift workers lose a lot of circadian nocturnal orientation during days off, but such steps should help to lessen some of the damage.

In conclusion, in thinking about biological clock strategies, shift workers should try to imagine themselves as the biological clock deep inside their head. We know when the body eats, lays down to sleep, exerts itself; we know when daylight is hitting our eyes and when things are loud and when things are quiet. Just where the biological clock decides to put 'night' and where to put 'day' will depend on the mixture of information that it receives from the various senses. The more consistent that information is, and the more regular it is over time, the easier and the quicker will be the readjustment process.

> **Box 8.3**
>
> From a single mother with a school-aged daughter who took a part-time night shift job to make ends meet.
>
> > I can only get a maximum of 6 hours sleep a day because of my responsibilities. In the mornings I take my daughter to school before going to bed. I also used to do the house cleaning then too, but had to stop that. Then, because I haven't unwound, I wake up constantly during the day because of listening out for things. In the afternoons I have to ferry my daughter around on the bus to ballet and tap classes and to see friends. I try to plan everything around not letting my daughter suffer because of my working. I do get irritable and snappy with her sometimes, though.

Social and domestic strategies

Ideally, the families of shift workers should be just as involved in acquiring the information presented in this book as the shift workers themselves. As we have discussed in Chapter 3, social and domestic problems affect everyone in the shift workers's family (Walker, 1985). Solutions and strategies must, therefore, come from the whole family. Few of the coping strategies outlined for the other two factors of the triad will work unless the social and domestic milieu is supportive. As an important first step, shift workers should seek to gain their family's understanding of their predicament and to rally their support in coping with it. Essentially the shift worker's family must be made aware that the overall coping strategy involves them in a very real way. There will be need for self-discipline, communication and sacrifice. Without that involvement the coping strategy will not work, and the family itself will be the victim of the resulting strife. Relationships should be forged with other shift work families who are more likely than day working friends to be supportive and understanding. Self-help groups can be extremely useful.

From a practical point of view, the first task for the family is to protect the shift worker from noise and commitments during the time that he or she has to sleep. The family must adopt the attitude that those times should be just as protected and free from commitments as are the night hours of day workers. It is simply not fair on the shift worker to expect him or her to interrupt their major sleep episode in order to fulfil some family or domestic commitment which could just as easily be carried out by another individual or at a different time of day.

The family should also make some purchases; they should buy heavy curtains or blinds for the shift worker's bedroom, a set of earplugs, and perhaps a thick pile carpet to deaden the sound around the bedroom (Monk, 1988). Some source of gentle white noise may help deaden some of the intrusive sounds coming from outside the bedroom window. Fortunately, technology has enabled television programmes to be recorded, while the use of walkmans or earphones can help to eliminate much of the noise that needs to occur in a household. All of these technologies should be adopted and strict family taboos should be invoked regarding noise during the sleep episode. Telephones should be replaced with ones where the ringer can be totally switched off, and front doorbells adjusted so they can be disconnected or switched off. An important rule to remember is: 'If the only person at home is a shift worker trying to sleep, there is no one at home'.

Attitudes, too, have to change. All family members should make considerable efforts to avoid requiring the shift worker to shorten or change the timing of his or her sleep. They should be tough with delivery men, they should reschedule doctors' appointments and shopping trips, friends should be warned about calling during the sleep time. Clearly it will not work 100% of the time, but there is usually much room for improvement. If everyone in the family knows when the sleep time is, arrangements are much easier to enforce. This, again, relates to the importance of regularity in the shift worker's sleep/wake routine. Other social and domestic coping strategies relate to the flow of information. The family should purchase a large monthly planner calendar of the type used in business, and put it up on the kitchen wall, marking the dates of that month on which the shift worker will be working days, evenings and nights. During each run of night work a sign should be put up reminding the family of the quiet times when the shift worker will be trying to sleep. Communication is vitally important, and the shift worker should actively try and make sure that the spouse and other family members understand some of the problems and concerns that are on their mind. It can often be helpful to direct anger and frustration at the shift work situation itself, rather than at other family members. In that way the family can unite in being anti-shift work, rather than fighting amongst themselves while the real culprit is the unnatural routine that the shift worker is being asked to work (Box 8.4).

> **Box 8.4**
>
> From a 33-year-old married security officer, wife works part-time, two children at school. Irregular shifts.
>
> I feel irritable. I'm almost ashamed to admit it, but I do tend to get argumentative if I miss out on sleep and unfortunately I take it out on my wife and children which I know isn't fair. At the time, when I start arguing I just can't be doing with them around me and I'm saying 'You'll have to wait a minute', I start snapping at them. I think I shouldn't have done that, and I feel guilty afterwards, but at the time it's just so spontaneous that you feel as though you can't help yourself. In actual fact we have arguments because we have arguments, if you know what I mean. I'll feel tired and I'll start snapping at the children. Or I'll start at the wife and she'll say 'There is no need to shout at me like that' or 'There's no need to be like that with the children' and I'll say 'well I know there isn't but you know I've just been on nights and I just can't be doing with people around me at that time'.

Time should be reserved for various activities which will help in the communication process. The shift worker should not just set aside time for sleep, but also set aside time for being with the children, and for quiet time alone with his or her spouse. The shift worker should remember that these activities are much more important than painting the garage or doing the shopping. Of course, such domestic chores have to be done, and time should be set aside to do them in, but it is important not to let that time eat into the time needed to spend with spouses and/or children (or indeed the time needed for sleep). Often, domestic chores can be used as an escape whereby the shift worker avoids having to interact with the family. This is a pathological response to the situation and one which will inevitably lead to a worsening of the situation. Very often, shift workers are seen who are obviously taking on other commitments, perhaps a moonlighting job or extra overtime, perhaps a hobby which is very demanding of time, purely as a means of escaping some of the interpersonal tensions that are there in the family. Such strategies only delay the inevitable social and emotional disaster that will eventually affect the whole family. This is particularly important when considering extra weekend work or overtime (Box 8.5). The obvious advantages of earning more money need to be offset against the less obvious costs to family and

Box 8.5

From a furnace man on a regular 4-week rota.

> I am a member of a local shooting club and not having weekends interferes with my social life and hobbies. I have to be told about social events well in advance so that I can weigh up whether to go or not. Saturday and Friday are very profitable overtime shifts which I do not want to miss, but they clash with my social life. I also swap shifts with a colleague so that I work weekends, allowing me to attend adult education classes mid week.
>
> I never see my 17-year-old daughter. She is always out although I have asked her to stay in more in the evenings. I would see her more if I worked days as she was usually in the house until 7 pm and at weekends. However, I only have 13 weekends off a year and these are often taken up with overtime.

social life. A balance needs to be struck between a rich family and a happy one!

As we have said throughout this book, shift work is a source of stress. Stress can either be invigorating, bringing out the best in a group of people, or destructive, tearing the group apart. If the family is to cope successfully with shift work it will be because it faced up to it, recognized the needs and challenges, and lived up to them, rather than denying the needs and challenges and running away from them. The family working together forcefully and rationally to cope with shift work can only gain in cohesiveness and strength.

Beating fatigue at work

Introduction

The major aim of this book has been to improve the biological and social coping strategies of the shift worker so that he or she does not appear at work in a 'zombie-like' state. Shift work is too broad and multifaceted a problem to be solvable exclusively by worktime interventions. The positioning of this section after discussion of those more general, and arguably more important, strategies is thus deliberate. The fact remains, however, that sleepiness at work is bound to remain a significant safety problem in all but the most successfully adjusted employee. The aim of this section is to develop specific strategies at work and on the journey home, which will reduce that risk. These strategies should of course be used in addition to the shift work coping strategies outlined earlier in this chapter.

At the end of an evening shift

Studies of circadian rhythms and sleep patterns of evening shift workers have revealed few problems. For example, Professor Knauth and his colleagues (1980) have found that evening shift workers sleep significantly longer than either day shift or night shift workers. Similarly, studies of circadian rhythms in evening shift workers have found that they continue to exhibit robust circadian variation (Kogi,

1985). The problem areas regarding fatigue for evening shift workers are during the last one or two hours of the shift, and on the drive home in the early hours of the morning. Such problems will hit particularly hard if the shift worker happens to be a morning type person who likes to be 'up with the dawn' (see Chapter 7). The most important thing not to do on the evening shift is to take caffeine. Although it would indeed help in the short term, inevitably on the evening shift the individual will be trying to sleep within a couple of hours of finishing work and there will thus be extra problems occurring during that sleep which will far outweigh any short-term gains. Rather, evening shift workers should try to keep active during the last few hours of the shift. They should be encouraged to move around, to talk to other people, and to save up their rest breaks for that time. If possible, work should be scheduled so that the monotonous and boring tasks come earlier in the evening shift and the more interesting tasks later on in the shift. Workers should be encouraged to get into the routine of having a fruit juice or decaffeinated drink an hour before the end of the shift; this will serve as a milestone that makes that last hour seem to pass a little less slowly. As we shall discuss in the next chapter, employers should make sure that decaffeinated beverages and the availability of a hearty evening meal are there for their evening shift workers.

Evening shift workers should be very careful indeed on their way home from work. They are in a very high risk situation. First, they are tired, with the circadian systems starting to shut down various functions in anticipation of sleep. Secondly, it is dark and traffic accidents are 33% more likely to occur in darkness than in daylight. Third, many of the people with whom they are sharing the road may be drunk. Evening shift workers on their way home should drive very defensively, expecting every other road user to be a drunk driver, giving them a wide birth and anticipating irritating and/or irrational driving. The car interior should be kept cool with some lively music or talk on the radio to keep the driver from nodding off to sleep at the wheel. Varying the route home, and making a point of noticing things on the route, can be very effective ways of beating fatigue.

While we are considering the journey home we would also advise against stopping off for a late night drink to unwind. There are a number of reasons besides traffic safety why this is not a good idea. First, it is making the change in the biological clock timing greater, i.e. worse, than it has to be. If the shift worker goes to bed at 1.30 am all he or she has to contend with is a couple of hours' difference from a normal day worker's sleep. Spend an extra couple of hours in a bar or night club, and one has to turn oneself into a night worker, not getting to bed until almost dawn. Secondly, as we have discussed earlier, alcohol is not good for sleep; it fragments the sleep resulting in sleep that is lighter and shorter in duration.

Coping with the night shift

Although things are bad at the end of an evening shift usually they're downright awful in the last half of a night of 'graveyard' shift (Box 8.6). However well the shift worker is doing with coping measures, the hours around 4 to 6 am are bound to be the most difficult in terms of trying to remain awake. Figure 8.2 shows some data we collected (with Dr David Embrey) of shift working process controllers at a large chemical plant. By studying them at work for a whole month we obtained temperature and subjective alertness ratings around the clock. The 4am slump is quite visible. As we have discussed in Chapter 2, there are sound biological reasons for that difficulty. What, though, can the individual do in order to combat it?

> **Box 8.6**
>
> From a 46-year-old male print room supervisor on rotating shifts 90 nights a year. Two teenage children. Wife part-time teacher.
>
> It's a critical time 6–7 in the morning. Once you've past that stage you're OK. That's the really critical time. If I sit down for one minute between 6–7 am I'll go to sleep. I've never done it before except once. If we're busy, we're busy and we do not have time for cat-napping but if there is a slack period I tend to walk about the building and go and talk to the security guards, take a breath of fresh air and come back. That's the time when you tend to make a lot of mistakes. If you're trying so hard but it's not happening you make mistakes. You try hard not to sleep and that's when you can't help but make mistakes.

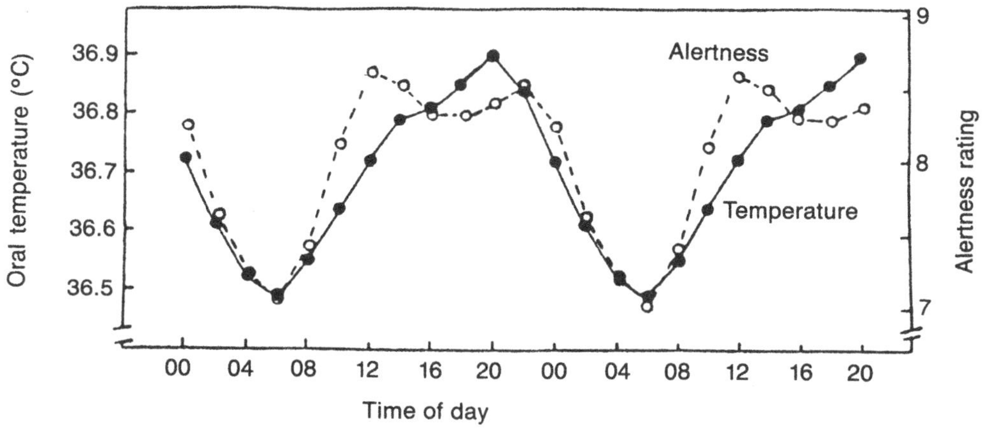

Figure 8.2 Circadian rhythms in oral temperature and subjective alertness in a group of six rapidly rotating shift workers studied over a month. Readings were only taken while at work (after Monk and Embrey, 1981).

First, a little caffeine may help if that is what the individual is used to. A few cups of coffee or cans of cola might help the individual to remain alert and vigilant. It is vitally important, though, that the caffeine be taken prior to 3am, otherwise the caffeine will still be in the bloodstream when the shift worker is trying to sleep at home. Second, the shift should, if possible, be structured with strategically placed rest breaks and meal breaks. Shift workers should avoid the situation in which a long, unbroken session of work stretches in front of them, particularly in the early hours of the morning. Ideally it should be possible for them to take a short break to walk around, get something to drink and eat or use the bathroom every two hours or so.

It is also important that the night shift worker takes a proper lunch break halfway through the shift. The more normal this lunch break is the better. Again, technology can help by enabling the provision of microwave cookers or vending machines, so that the night shift workers can have a hot lunch halfway through their work period. Social activities during that break should also be encouraged; there is no reason why the night shift lunch should not have as many activities going on as does the day shift equivalent. The 4 am slump will then be that much easier to take.

Unless the shift worker is on a rapidly rotating shift system (or is really desperate) it is probably best for them not to sleep during the lunch break of the night shift. There are two reasons for this; first, it will confuse the circadian system into thinking it is still alright to sleep at night; secondly, there is sleep inertia. Sleep inertia is the grogginess people feel after being woken up after a short sleep. Studies find that sleep inertia is particularly bad at 4 am (Naitoh, 1981), so a nap then might reduce safety. Operating dangerous machinery while suffering from sleep inertia is not something to be recommended!

As with the evening shift, if they are able to, night shift workers should try to reschedule their work so that the monotonous and boring tasks do not hit them at the time when their will to stay awake is at its weakest. They should recognize, too, that their abilities will not be the same all the way through the shift. If possible, they should try to avoid scheduling particularly dangerous or critical operations at or near the 4 to 6 am slump. As we shall see in the following chapter, improvements in the environment can also help. The employer should consider providing good bright lighting, comfortable heat levels and a generally stimulating environment for the worker.

Following the night shift is the journey home. Here the night worker is still at risk but more from himself or herself than from others. Few drunk drivers are on the road and at least it will probably be daylight now. The individual's alertness will not be total, however, and he or she should be sure still to drive defensively and use some of the tricks mentioned earlier in order to keep alert.

Feasting and fasting diets

In the late 1970s, work by Dr Ehret (1981) and colleagues, based on studies using laboratory rats, suggested that an elaborate ritual of feasting on some days, fasting on others and drinking precisely timed cups of strong black coffee could help the human biological clock adjust more quickly to a change in routine. It was tried among other countermeasures in a jet-lag study with some positive results (Graeber, *et al.*, 1981). Since then there has been quite a lot of publicity regarding it, some heralding it as a panacea for the shift work and jet-lag situations. However, many experts disagree with the basic premise of this countermeasure and even those who were involved in the jet-lag study purportedly confirming its benefits, have doubts about the worth of the feasting and fasting manipulation (Graeber, 1989). As in many other situations the problem here is one of a possible placebo effect, whereby any ritual or possible cure can, just by the act of doing something, make people feel that it is working. When the novelty wears off, the countermeasure loses all effectiveness. We cannot be sure how much of the beneficial effects of the feasting and fasting diet may be due to placebo effects. Other special countermeasures will undoubtedly be suggested in the future. Before investing too much time and money in them, care should be taken to ensure that they have been properly tested over time, and are not simply placebo effects which disappear after a few months.

Medication and drug therapies

Since one of the major complaints of shift workers is that they obtain insufficient sleep, an obvious countermeasure is to improve that sleep by the use of hypnotic medication (sleeping pills). There are two major problems with medication use, one of which has been solved, the other not.

The first problem with using hypnotics to improve daytime sleeps is that of 'residual' or 'carry-over' effects which leave the worker still drowsy in the evening and night when he or she needs to be alert. Such effects (which are characteristic of the barbiturates and longer-acting hypnotics) can exacerbate the sleepiness due to circadian effects (see above) leading to a potentially dangerous situation for the worker (Buysse, 1991). These problems have been overcome to some extent by the development of short-acting benzodiazepines such as triazolam (marketed as Halcion R), which have a half-life of only a few hours (Seidel *et al.*, 1984). In a 1984 St Louis study, Dr Walsh and colleagues (1984) showed that fairly large (0.5 mg) doses of triazolam did indeed significantly improve the day sleep of night workers. Importantly, though, this did not appear to result in any increased phase adjustment of the circadian clock relative to placebo. Thus after two nights of the drug, day sleeps 3 and 4 (with placebo) were no better than for those who had received placebo all the way through. Putative phase resetting properties of large doses of triazolam in hamsters (Turek and Losee-Olson, 1986) now appear to have been due to the changes in the activity patterns of the animals, rather than to anything more profound.

The second problem regarding the use of hypnotics by shift workers has most definitely not been solved, and is the reason why hypnotics are not recommended for this group (Monk, 1989). It relates to the chronic nature of the shift worker's problem. There has yet to be a hypnotic which is recommended for anything other than occasional transient insomnia. The shift worker's insomnia is frequent and chronic and the dual problems of tolerance and dependence imply that shift workers using hypnotics on a regular basis are probably deriving little or no benefit from them. Instead, they are being deceived into thinking such drugs are effective by the 'rebound insomnia' they experience upon withdrawal of the drug. Moreover, chronic high doses of triazolam have in some cases been associated with mood changes, an effect to which shift workers are especially vulnerable (Adam and Oswald, 1989). Until hypnotics are developed which are totally benign in the chronic administration condition, it is infeasible that shift workers can achieve any lasting benefit from such drugs.

Although a hypnotic may, in the short term, improve a shift worker's sleep, what is truly needed is a 'chronobiotic' (Simpson *et al.*, 1973) which will facilitate the resetting of his or her circadian system. Although various substances have been touted as chronobiotics the evidence is far from conclusive, and Professor Alain Reinberg (Reinberg *et al.*, 1987) speaks for many experts in concluding that a true chronobiotic has yet to be discovered. Apart from those drugs which are suspect because of their hypnotic properties (e.g. the benzodiazepines) which might render the phase shift more apparent than real, the prime candidate has been theophylline. Although there is some evidence of chronobiotic properties in rodents (Ehret *et al.*, 1975), in man the results have been negative, both in carefully controlled experiments at NASA-Ames, and in view of the fact that 'millions of asthmatic patients consume rather large doses of theophylline daily to avert bronchospasm without complaining of jet-lag symptoms' (Reinberg *et al.*, 1987). It would therefore seem premature to assert that this drug has chronobiotic properties which would be of benefit to shift workers.

The oral administration of melatonin as a phase shift countermeasure does hold some promise in view of the obvious role of the hormone in the human circadian system. Dr Josephine Arendt's team recently tried melatonin as a countermeasure in a small jet-lag study with some success, predominantly in subjective measures of 'jet-lag' and in circadian cortisol rhythms. No beneficial effects were found in body temperature or performance, however (Arendt *et al.*, 1986; Arendt *et al.*, 1987).

Conclusions

From the above discussion it is clear that there definitely are things that the shift worker can do in order to ameliorate his or her shift working problem. However, there is no single panacea or 'quick fix' to shift work problems. Rather, it would appear that the individual must battle with the problems of shift work on a number of different fronts related to sleep, the circadian system, the social and domestic situation, as well as actual behaviour on the job that serves to keep the individual alert and vigilant through the shift hours.

References

Adam, K. and Oswald, I. (1989) Can a rapidly eliminated hypnotic cause daytime anxiety? *Pharmacopsychiatry*, **22**, 115–119.

Arendt, J., Aldhous, M. and Marks, V. (1986) Alleviation of jet-lag by melatonin: Preliminary results of a controlled double blind trial. *Br. Med. J.*, **292**, 1170.

Arendt, J., Minors, D.S. and Waterhouse, J.M., (1989) Basic concepts and implications. In *Biological Rhythms in Clinical Practice*, edited by Arendt, J., Minors, D.S. and Waterhouse, J.M., pp. 3–7, London: Wright.

Arendt, J.H., Aldhous, M., English, J., Marks, V., Marks, M. and Folkard, S. (1987) Some effects of jet-lag and their alleviation by melatonin. *Ergonomics*, **30**, 1379–1393.

Aschoff, J., Hoffman, K., Pohl, H. and Wever, R.A. (1975) Re-entrainment of circadian rhythms after phase-shifts of the zeitgeber. *Chronobiologia*, **2**, 23–78.

Buysse, D.J. (1991) Drugs affecting sleep, sleepiness and performance. In *Sleep, Sleepiness and Performance*, edited by Monk, T.H., pp. 249–306, Chichester: John Wiley & Sons.

Czeisler, C.A., Moore-Ede, M.C. and Coleman, R.M. (1982) Rotating shift work schedules that disrupt sleep are improved by applying circadian principles. *Science*, **217**, 460–463.

Czeisler, C.A., Allan, J.S., Strogatz, S.H. *et al.* (1986) Bright light resets the human circadian pacemaker independent of the timing of the sleep–wake cycle. *Science*, **233**, 667–671.

Czeisler, C.A., Johnson, M.P., Duffy, J.F., Brown, E.N., Ronda, J.M. and Kronauer, R.E. (1990) Exposure to bright light and darkness to treat physiologic maladaptation to night work. *N. Engl. J. Med.*, **322**, 1253–1259.

Dorsey, C.M. (1991) Failing to sleep: psychological and behavioral underpinnings of insomnia. In *Sleep, Sleepiness and Performance*, edited by Monk, T.H., pp. 223–248, Chichester: John Wiley & Sons.

Eastman, C.I. (1987) Bright light in work–sleep schedules for shift workers: Application of circadian rhythm principles. In *Temporal Disorder in Human Oscillatory Systems*, edited by Rensing, L., van der Heiden, U. and Mackey, M.C., pp. 176–185, New York: Springer-Verlag.

Ehret, C.F., (1981) New approaches to chronohygiene for the shift worker in the nuclear power industry. In *Night and Shift Work: Biological and Social Aspects*, edited by Reinberg, A., Vieux, N. and Andlauer, P., pp. 263–270, Oxford: Pergamon Press.

Ehret, C.F., Potter, V.R. and Dobra, K.W. (1975) Chronotypic action of theophylline and of pentabarbital as circadian zeitgebers in the rat. *Science*, **188**, 1212–1215.

Graeber, R.C. (1989) Jet lag and sleep disruption. In *Principles and Practice of Sleep Medicine*, edited by Kryger, M.H., Roth, T. and Dement, W.C., pp. 324–331, Philadelphia: W.B. Saunders Company.

Graeber, R.C., Sing, H.C. and Cuthbert, B.N. (1981) The impact of transmeridian flight on deploying soldiers. In *Variations in Work–Sleep Schedules: Effects on Health and Performance*, 7th edn, edited by Johnson, L.C., Tepas, D.I., Colquhoun, W.P. and Colligan, M.J., pp. 513–537, New York: Spectrum: Advances in Sleep Research.

Hauri, P.J. (1983) A cluster analysis of insomnia. *Sleep*, **6**(4), 326–338.

Horne, J.A. (1988) *Why We Sleep: the Functions of Sleep in Humans and Other Mammals*, Oxford: Oxford University Press.

Ilmarinen, J., Ilmarinen, R., Korhonen, O. and Nurminen, M. (1980) Circadian variation of physiological functions related to physical work capacity. *Scand. J. Work Environ. Health*, **6**, 112–122.

Knauth, P., Landau, K., Droge, C., Schwitteck, M., Widynski, M. and Rutenfranz, J. (1980) Duration of sleep depending on the type of shift work. *Int. Arch. Occup. Environ. Health*, **46**, 167–177.

Kogi, K. (1985) Introduction to the problems of shift work. In *Hours of Work – Temporal Factors in Work Scheduling*, edited by Folkard, S. and Monk, T.H., pp. 165–184, New York: John Wiley & Sons.

Lewy, A.J., Wehr, T.A., Goodwin, F.K., Newsome, D.A. and Markey, S.P. (1980) Light suppresses melatonin secretion in humans. *Science*, **210**, 1267–1269.

Monk, T.H. (1986) Advantages and disadvantages of rapidly rotating shift schedules – A circadian viewpoint. *Hum. Factors*, **28**, 553–557.

Monk, T.H. (1988a) Coping with the stress of shift work. *Work and Stress*, **2**, 169–172.

Monk, T.H. (1988b) *How to Make Shift Work Safe and Productive*, Des Plaines, Ill. American Society of Safety Engineers.

Monk, T.H. (1989) Shift work. In *Principles and Practice of Sleep Medicine*, edited by Kryger, M.H., Roth, T. and Dement, W.C., pp. 332–337, Philadelphia: W.B. Saunders Company.

Monk, T.H. and Embrey, D.E. (1981) A field study of circadian rhythms in actual and interpolated task performance. In *Night and Shift Work: Biological and Social Aspects*, edited by Reinberg, A., Vieux, N. and Andlauer, P., pp.473–480, Oxford: Pergamon Press.

Naitoh, P. (1981) Circadian cycles and restorative power of naps. In *The Twenty-four Hour Workday*, Publication #81–127, edited by Johnson, L.C., Tepas, D.I., Colquhoun, W.P. and Colligan, M.J., pp. 693–720, Cincinnati, OH: Department of Health and Human Services (NIOSH).

Reinberg, A., Smolensky, M. and Labrecque, G. (1987) The hunting of a wonder pill for resetting all biological clocks. *Annu. Rev. Chronopharmacol.*, **4**, 171–208.

Seidel, W.F., Roth, T., Roehrs, T., Zorick, F. and Dement, W.C. (1984) Treatment of a 12-hour shift of sleep schedule with benzodiazepines. *Science*, **224**, 1262–1264 (Abstract).

Simpson, H.W., Bellamy, N., Bohlen, J. and Halberg, F. (1973) Double blind trial of a possible chronobiotic: Quiadon. *Int. J. Chronobiol.*, **1**, 287–311.

Turek, F.W. and Losee-Olson, S. (1986) A benzodiazepine used in the treatment of insomnia phase-shifts the mammalian circadian clock. *Nature*, **321**, 167–168.

Van Loon, J.H. (1963) Diurnal body temperature curves in shift workers. *Ergonomics*, **6**, 267–272.

Walker, J.M. (1985) Social problems of shift work. In *Hours of Work – Temporal Factors in Work Scheduling*, edited by Folkard, S. and Monk, T.H., pp. 211–225, New York: John Wiley & Sons.

Walsh, J.K., Muehlbach, M.J. and Scweitzer, P.K. (1984) Acute administration of triazolam for the daytime sleep of rotating shift workers. *Sleep*, **7**, 223–229.

Wever, R.A. (1979) *The Circadian System of Man: Results of Experiments Under Temporal Isolation*, New York: Springer-Verlag.

Wever, R.A., Poiasek, J. and Wildgruber, C.M. (1983) Bright light affects human circadian rhythms. *Pflugers Arch.*, **396**, 85–87.

Yules, R.B., Freedman, D.X. and Chandler, K.A. (1966) The effect of ethyl alcohol on man's electroencephalographic sleep cycle. *Electroencephalogr. Clin. Neurophysiol.*, **20**, 109–111.

Chapter 9

Strategies for the employer

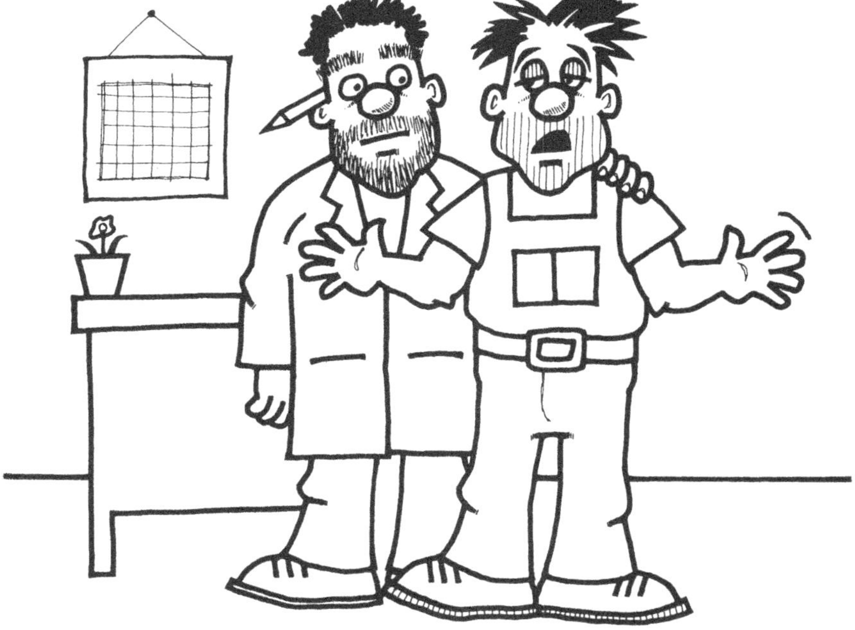

Introduction

Although there are certain things an individual shift worker can do about improving his or her situation, in many areas the individual is unable to act, and must rely upon interventions from the company or organization for which he or she works. Thus, although the timing of sleep/wake routines, attention to diet, management of zeitgebers and adoption of a social/domestic strategy all fall within the remit of the individual shift worker, the selection of shift schedules, manipulation of environmental conditions, employee selection and job specification usually all fall to the employer. Unfortunately, the employer seldom takes this responsibility seriously. Unless required otherwise by legislation, employers are often content to muddle along with poorly conceived ad hoc solutions used simply from habit. Very often the attitude of management is either 'If it ain't broke don't fix it' if the problems are not immediately apparent, and 'don't fan the flames' if they are. A genuine learning process is often needed by senior management if these counterproductive attitudes are to be overcome.

Management education

The first major breakthrough required in management education is to convince a company's senior decision makers that a more enlightened approach to shift work will almost certainly save the company money, making it more productive and competitive. As hiring, selection and training costs rise, it can make strong economic sense to have a contented and well-coping shift workforce, as opposed to a poorly coping one with high turnover and absenteeism rates. Sometimes management fear that the organization will be forced into a radical restructuring of their whole shift working operation along 'chronobiological principles'. This is an unfortunate perception; very often significant benefits can be gained with intermediate steps involving employee education and support services.

As in many other areas, the ultimate sanction against indifference in management to shift worker problems may be the legal one. It may well be that litigation from sick or injured shift workers becomes the means by which perceived harm is recompensed. Any worker taking that route would have no shortage of expert testimony to support the argument that shift work practices are by and large harmful. In 1979, for example, The Shift Work Committee at Japan's Association of Industrial Health (1979) stated '. . . in particular, the introduction of shiftwork for economic reasons related to accelerated depreciation of costly machinery or managerial efficiency must be prohibited'. From the United States, Professor Tepas and his colleagues (1981) have remarked that 'Night work might prove to be an insidious silent killer'. It is a sobering exercise to compare the different legislative attitudes to shift work current in the UK and the US as compared with the rest of the world. This is particularly true for women (Singer, 1989) who are prohibited from night work (with certain exceptions) in many other countries (e.g. Belgium, Czechoslovakia, France, Germany, Italy, the Netherlands and Norway). Moreover, even when night work is not prohibited, legislation exists regarding hours in the working week (France [39 hours], Brazil [36 hours]) and medical officer coverage (Austria). Indeed the entire European community (EC) is currently considering a proposed directive that would limit night work hours and mandate at least 11 hours of off duty between shifts.

Prosaically, one reason for the relative simplicity of many shift systems, and their continued retention, despite being chronobiologically unsound, is that they have been put together by middle or lower-level supervisors with few intellectual or information processing resources available to help them. Recently, with the advent of personal computers and scheduling programs, it has become more feasible to move away from the more simplistic approaches. Some authors (Schwarzenau *et al.*, 1986) have developed a shift schedule selection procedure involving computer programs that enhance the most chronobiologically acceptable features.

Shift work schedules

For the employer, the major advance made by the scientific study of human circadian rhythms has been the information it has provided regarding the suitability or otherwise of various shift work schedules. The most important information concerns the slow rate of re-entrainment (phase adjustment) of the circadian system to a change in routine, requiring more than a week to phase adjust to night work (Monk *et al.*, 1978). This is covered extensively in Chapter 2 (see Figure 2.7 for example).

Also important (again, as discussed in Chapter 2) is the direction of phase shift that is being attempted. The human biological clock has a natural tendency to run slow, with a preferred period of around 25 hours, rather than the 24 hours of nature and society (Wever, 1979).

Thus, under free-running conditions, bedtimes become progressively later by about one hour per day, a phenomenon confirmed by a tendency for people to go to bed later on weekends, rather than earlier. Perhaps because of this tendency to 'run slow', the human circadian system appears to phase adjust more slowly to phase advances (60 minutes of phase changed per day) than to phase delays (90 minutes of phase change per day) (Aschoff *et al.*, 1975; Klein *et al.*, 1972). This suggests that shift rotation in the clockwise direction (mornings, then evenings, then nights) would be easier to cope with than rotation in the counter-clockwise direction (nights then evenings then mornings). Although that prediction still needs to be properly tested in the field, there is some supportive evidence for it (Czeisler *et al.*, 1982).

There are a multitude of different shift schedules currently in use. Many approximate a 'weekly rotation' whereby an employee works between four and seven shifts at one timing before changing to another. This is particularly disheartening because most shift work experts agree that from a chronobiological point of view, weekly rotation is the speed of rotation that is the most likely to produce problems (Czeisler *et al.*, 1982; Akerstedt *et al.*, 1977; Rutenfranz *et al.*, 1977; Smith, 1979). Thus, while there is insufficient time for the biological clock to realign completely to the new temporal orientation, there is enough time to build up a sizeable sleep debt (Tilley *et al.*, 1982). Between them, the circadian desynchronosis and partial sleep deprivation will inevitably result in malaise and on the job performance decrements.

Having decided upon the shift system or rota to avoid, it is less easy to decide upon the optimum alternative to select. Expert opinion here is divided. Most European and Scandinavian experts (Rutenfranz *et al.*, 1977) favour rapid rotation with very short (1- or 2-day) rounds of duty at one shift timing before moving to a different timing. In contrast, North American experts (Czeisler *et al.*, 1982; Moore-Ede and Richardson, 1985) favour much slower rotation speeds, with three weeks or more at one shift timing before moving to a different timing. The controversy is discussed elsewhere in detail (Monk, 1986); essentially it revolves around the loss of nocturnal orientation during 'weekend breaks' (Van Loon, 1963), and the relative levels of harm considered to be induced by 'inappropriate phasing' (having to work when the body and brain are geared to sleep) as compared with 'circadian dissociation' (the breakdown in the harmony of all the various rhythmic processes).

One approach to resolving the issue is to consider the task the shift worker is being asked to perform. Different tasks not only show different 'best' times during the circadian cycle, but also phase adjust at different rates to a change in routine (Folkard and Monk, 1979; Monk and Folkard, 1985). Highly cognitive tasks involving working memory, mental calculations and verbal reasoning appear to peak earlier in the day and to phase adjust more quickly than the more simple repetitive or 'automatic' tasks such as driving, quality control and monitoring.

In terms of performance demands, unadjusted (i.e. diurnally orientated) night workers are likely to find tasks involving serial search, inspection and/or the maintenance of vigilance (e.g. driving) to be particularly disrupted. Ample opportunity for, and circadian countermeasures designed to encourage, circadian re-alignment should thus be concentrated on such workers. Shift rotation speed should be slow in the phase delay direction, so that a nocturnal orientation can be rapidly acquired and maintained (Czeisler *et al.*, 1982). Shift workers should be counselled to use sleep schedules and time cues (zeitgebers) which will aid this process. In contrast, tasks involving immediate retention and high memory loads will be performed relatively well during the night shift, even in diurnally orientated individuals (Monk and Embrey, 1981). In these cases, therefore, rapidly rotating shift systems (e.g. the 'Metropolitan rota' of two mornings, two evenings, two nights and two days off) might be a suitable alternative. In such systems the circadian system retains its diurnal orientation, and a gradual build-up of sleep loss over a long run of night duty is avoided (Tilley *et al.*, 1982). Whichever alternative schedule is selected, it should be remembered that there is now hard empirical evidence that significant improvements can accrue from a move away from a weekly rotating schedule, be it to a more slowly (Czeisler *et al.*, 1982) or more rapidly (Williamson and Sanderson, 1986; Knauth and Kiesswetter, 1987) rotating system.

Bright lights at the workplace

Throughout the 1960s and 1970s, the dominant view of the human circadian system was that it was largely unaffected by light/dark cycles except in as much as they influenced patterns of behaviour (Wever, 1979). However, Lewy and colleagues' (1980) demonstration that only daylight levels of illumination were sufficient to suppress endogenous melatonin production at night, opened up a whole new set of studies using daylight (> 2000 Lux) levels of illumination in time isolation studies which had previously been concerned with comparatively dim artificial light.

The hormone melatonin is produced in the pineal and has been shown to be associated with tiredness when circulating in the bloodstream (Akerstedt *et al.*, 1982). Thus, its suppression was thought to be important to the circadian system. Laboratory studies in both West Germany (Wever, 1988) and the United States (Czeisler *et al.*, 1986; 1989) have confirmed that bright lights can be extremely powerful as resetting agents (zeitgebers) of the human circadian system. Professor Wever (1988) has shown a dramatic increase in the range of entrainment (essentially equivalent to the 'hours of phase shift per day' rate) when bright lights are used to stretch or shrink circadian 'days'. Dr Czeisler and colleagues have shown in a 1986 Harvard University study that 3 days of evening bright light exposure can delay the phase of the circadian rhythms of a woman suffering from advance phase sleep syndrome. Dr Czeisler's group (Czeisler *et al.*, 1989) has also derived a human phase response curve to bright light (with room light levels factored in), which suggests that phase resetting in the laboratory can be accomplished in three days if the timing of the light is appropriate (and if competing zeitgebers are either absent or ineffectual).

A recent study by Czeisler and colleagues (1990) sought directly to test the efficacy of daylight levels of illumination (7000 to 12000 Lux) in the workplace of night workers, supplemented by rigid darkness enforcement during their (daytime) sleep episode. From both a study of night time alertness and performance and a determination of the phase (timing) of the circadian system, these countermeasures appeared significantly to help as compared with a 'laissez-faire', 'dim light (150 Lux) at work' control condition. Although the sample size was small and the subjects were not 'real' shift workers, the gains were impressive and hard to dispute. However, the controversy arises as to whether the phase resetting gains were achieved primarily because of the bright lights per se, or because of the behavioural modifications imposed by the specification of 8 hours of complete darkness (09.00 to 17.00) in the bedroom after working the night shift in the bright light condition (Van Cauter and Turek, 1990). We would favour the latter interpretation, asserting that it was facilitated (or perhaps, even, enabled) by the rises in nocturnal arousal and suppression of melatonin induced by the bright lights.

Applying bright light exposure therapy to shift workers has also been the concern of other investigators. By rigourous use of goggles, light-proofed bedrooms and banks of bright lights, Dr Charmane Eastman (1987) has shown that in some cases entrainment to non-24-hour routines can be attained by highly controlled bright light exposure. However, most recently she has concluded (Eastman, 1989) from a larger study that such procedures are at best partial in their success. This largely negative conclusion is echoed by Moline and colleagues (1989) finding that circadian rhythms in a simulated jet-lag study appeared to be, if anything, more disrupted by (post-shift) morning bright light exposure. Finally, there are cautions concerning possible retinal damage from chronic exposure to extremely bright artificial lights. Thus, while the theoretically-orientated laboratory studies of bright light re-entrainment in humans are important and intriguing, their precise practical application for the shift worker may take some time to work out.

Having described all the caveats, however, there are few experts who would disagree with the assertion that a bright, stimulating work environment is much better for a night worker than a dim and cozy one. Even if such stimulation does not actually phase reset the circadian system (and in rapidly rotating systems that might well prove to be counterproductive) it would certainly help overcome some of the losses in alertness that night work is heir to.

Clinical support

Clinical support specifically tailored for shift workers is only just starting to be developed. This is unfortunate because people would undoubtedly benefit from company 'shift work clinics' where physicians, chronobiologists, sleep clinicians and family therapists could be available to help those who are coping poorly. Such centres could be useful sources of information on coping strategies and medical referral (e.g. to family therapists, substance abuse treatment, etc.) and the major avenues for information flow regarding shift work. This would undoubtedly lower the level of strain experienced by the company's shift workers, even if the stress of the shift working routine remains the same.

Canteen and recreational resources

As well as providing medical and educational resources, employers should realize that the provision of canteen and recreational resources can be most helpful in enabling their shift workers to cope. Indeed some authors (although not the present ones) would follow the review of Dr Harrington (1978) in asserting that all of the gastro-intestinal problems reported by shift workers can be blamed on the poor dietary choices available to the shift worker. While we would emphasize the circadian dysfunction route to such problems, such problems would undoubtedly be lessened if proper canteen facilities were available. Similarly, problems of night shift absenteeism, tardiness and poor production will inevitably be exacerbated if such workers regard themselves as being treated like 'second-class citizens', denied access to recreational activities and events made available to the day working majority.

Shift work awareness programmes

As mentioned in previous chapters, much of the strain of shift work could be reduced by education and social support programmes which help employees to understand why they may be having problems, to reassure them that they are not weak, sick or in a bad marriage, and to help them to begin to develop their own personal solutions. The exact form that such a 'Shift Work Awareness Programme' (SWAP) would take would depend to a large extent upon who is implementing it. Both medical and safety departments of large organizations can be ideal developers and implementers of SWAPs, since both hold positions of trust for the employees, removed slightly from the 'us versus them' confrontational front line, and are well experienced in educational campaigns. Since shift work is both a medical and a safety issue, the practitioners involved should have no problem in justifying the presence of such a campaign within their department, although they will inevitably emphasize their own particular aspect of relevance.

In other situations the developer and implementer of the SWAP will be either an external consultant team, brought in by the company from outside the organization, or an internal consultant team recruited on an ad hoc basis from within the organization. In either case, a 'middle ground' must be found between the SWAP implementers and senior management with regard to the extent to which the SWAP will have an impact on the way the organization does its business.

Much of this book has been spent outlining the various problems connected with shift work. As always, it is easier to define problems than solutions and we have argued earlier that the shift work literature can be criticized for spending too much time on the former and too little on the latter. Any SWAP initiative must be sure to avoid the same trap. Moreover, a balance must be struck between the Utopian ideals of the scientist and the profit motive of the entrepreneur. Thus, for example, Professor Rutenfranz's (Rutenfranz *et al.*, 1977) assertion that at least 24 hours of free time must follow each night shift and Professor Kogi's 1985 assertion that shift work should not be introduced for purely economic reasons may be perfectly justifiable, but would be totally unacceptable (rightly or wrongly) in many organizations. Likewise, researchers must restrain their enthusiasm for more exotic shift schedules (e.g. 25 or 26-hour days), dictated solely by the properties of the biological clock (Eastman, 1987), realizing that such schedules may be totally at variance with the social and domestic life that the shift worker leads outside the workplace and may thus be unworkable in practice. On the other hand, senior management should exhibit restraint too, realizing that there is a biological clock, that shift work can be harmful to some people's health and well-being, and that some measure of legislative restraint is definitely required. To sugar the pill, employers should be reminded that shift work related problems can be very expensive, and that productivity improvements can result from implementation of more chronobiologically sensible shift schedules, particularly when combined with an education drive within the workforce.

Since there is usually so much room for improvement in the shift work aspects of an organization's functioning, it is often worthwhile for the SWAP to be conservative at first, concentrating on management and employee education, and the development of support services and self-help groups. As well as ameliorating some of the worst of the problems, and showing that SWAP can indeed be beneficial to the organization, these steps can often be helpful in laying the ground work for future more radical interventions (e.g. regarding shift scheduling). The organization as a whole may be much more responsive to such interventions if preceded by an educational initiative than if suddenly sprung on the organization.

In formulating a SWAP it is clearly necessary to adopt the multifaceted approach that has characterized this whole book. Education must address both the basic principles, i.e. the shift worker's various problems, and all the specific countermeasures designed to ameliorate them. Thus, all eight of the preceding chapters should be used to provide material that is moulded specifically to the organization concerned.

Conclusions

In conclusion, it is clear that, for the employer, as it was for the employee, the approach must be a multifaceted one. Not only shift selection, but also workplace design, employee education and the provision of clinical and nutritional resources must be considered part of the countermeasure package. For senior management it is vital to realize that whatever the cost of that package, it will in the end save the organization money.

References

Akerstedt, T., Gillberg, M. and Wetterberg, L. (1982) The circadian covariation of fatigue and urinary melatonin. *Biol. Psychiatry*, **17**, 547–552.

Akerstedt, T., Froberg, J., Levi, L., Torsvall, L. and Zamore, K. (1977) Shiftwork and well-being. *Reports from the Laboratory for Clinical Stress Research*, **63b**.

Aschoff, J., Hoffman, K., Pohl, H. and Wever, R.A. (1975) Re-entrainment of circadian rhythms after phase-shifts of the zeitgeber. *Chronobiologia*, **2**, 23–78.

Czeisler, C.A., Moore-Ede, M.C. and Coleman, R.M. (1982) Rotating shift work schedules that disrupt sleep are improved by applying circadian principles. *Science*, **217**, 460–463.

Czeisler, C.A., Allan, J.S., Strogatz, S.H., Rhonda, J.M., Sanchez, R., Ries, C.D., Freitag, W.O., Richardson, G.S. and Kronauer, R.E. (1986) Bright light resets the human circadian pacemaker independent of the timing of the sleep–wake cycle. *Science*, **233**, 667–671.

Czeisler, C.A., Kronauer, R.W., Allan, J.S., Duffy, J.F., Jewett, M.E., Brown, E.N. and Ronda, J.M. (1989) Bright light induction of strong (Type 0) resetting of the human circadian pacemaker. *Science*, **244**, 1328–1333.

Czeisler, C.A., Johnson, M.P., Duffy, J.F., Brown, E.N., Ronda, J.M. and Kronauer, R.E. (1990) Exposure to bright light and darkness to treat physiologic maladaptation to night work. *N. Engl. J. Med.*, **322**, 1253–1259.

Eastman, C.I. (1987) Bright light in work–sleep schedules for shift workers: Application of circadian rhythm principles. In *Temporal Disorder in Human Oscillatory Systems*, edited by Rensing, L., van der Heiden, U. and Mackey, M.C., pp. 176–185, New York: Springer-Verlag.

Eastman, C.I. (1989) Circadian rhythms during gradually advancing and delaying bright light and sleep schedules. *Sleep Res.*, **18**, 418.

Folkard, S. and Monk, T.H. (1979) Shiftwork and performance. *Hum. Factors*, **21**, 483–492.

Harrington, M. (1978) *Shiftwork and Health: a critical review of the literature*. London: HMSO.

Klein, K.E., Wegmann, H.M. and Hunt, B.I. (1972) Desynchronization of body temperature and performance circadian rhythms as a result of out-going and homegoing transmerdian flights. *Aerospace Med.*, **43**(2), 119–132.

Knauth, P. and Rutenfranz, J. (1982) Development of criteria for the design of shiftwork systems. *J. Hum. Ergol.*, **11**(Suppl), 337–367.

Knauth, P. and Kiesswetter, E. (1987) A change from weekly to quicker shift rotations: A field study of discontinuous three-shift workers. *Ergonomics*, **30**, 1311–1321.

Kogi, K. (1985) Introduction to the problems of shiftwork.

In *Hours of work: Temporal Factors in Work-Scheduling*, edited by Folkard, S. and Monk, T.H., pp. 165–184, Chichester: John Wiley and Sons.

Lewy, A.J., Wehr, T.A., Goodwin, F.K., Newsome, D.A. and Markey, S.P. (1980) Light suppresses melatonin secretion in humans. *Science*, **210**, 1267–1269.

Moline, M.L., Pollak, C.P., Wagner, D.R., Lester, L.S., Salter, C.A. and Hirsch, E. (1989) Effects of bright light on sleep following an acute phase advance. *Sleep Res.*, **18**, 432.

Monk, T.H. (1986) Advantages and disadvantages of rapidly rotating shift schedules – A circadian viewpoint. *Hum. Factors*, **28**, 553–557.

Monk, T.H. and Embrey, D.E. (1981) A field study of circadian rhythms in actual and interpolated task performance. In *Night and Shift Work: Biological and Social Aspects*, edited by Reinberg, A., Vieux, N. and Andlauer, P., pp. 473–480, Oxford: Pergamon Press.

Monk, T.H. and Folkard, S. (1985) Shiftwork and performance. In *Hours of Work – Temporal Factors in Work Scheduling*, edited by Folkard, S. and Monk, T.H., pp. 239–252, New York: John Wiley & Sons.

Monk, T.H., Knauth, P., Folkard, S. and Rutenfranz, J. (1978) Memory based performance measures in studies of shiftwork. *Ergonomics*, **21**, 819–826.

Moore-Ede, M.C. and Richardson, G.S. (1985) Medical implications of shiftwork. *Annu. Rev. Med.*, **36**, 607–617.

Rutenfranz, J., Colquhoun, W.P., Knauth, P. and Ghata, J.N. (1977) Biomedical and psychosocial aspects of shift work: A review. *Scand. J. Work. Environ. Health*, **3**, 165–182.

Schwarzenau, P., Knauth, P., Kiesswetter, E., Brockmann, W. and Rutenfranz, J. (1986) Algorithms for the computerized construction of shift systems which meet ergonomic criteria. *Appl. Ergonomics*, **17**, 169–176.

Shift Work Committee: Japan Association of Industrial Health (1979) Opinion on night work and shift work. *J. Sci. Labour*, **55**, 1–55.

Singer, G. (1989) Women and shiftwork. In *Managing Shiftwork*, edited by Wallace, M., pp. 25–48, Bundoora, Australia: Brain-Behavior Research Institute.

Smith, P.A. (1979) A study of weekly and rapidly rotating shiftworkers. *Int. Arch. Occup. Environ. Health*, **43**, 211–220 (Abstract).

Tasto, D.L. and Colligan, M.J. (1978) *Health Consequences of Shiftwork*. Project URU-4426, Technical Report. Menlo Park, CA: Stanford Research Institute.

Tepas, D.I., Walsh, J.K. and Armstrong, D.R. (1981) Comprehensive study of the sleep of shift workers. In *The Twenty-four Hour Workday: Proceedings of a Symposium on Variations in Work–Sleep Schedules*, edited by Johnson, L.C., Tepas, D.I., Colquhoun, W.P. and Colligan, M.J, pp. 419–433, Cincinnati, OH: Department of Health and Human Services (NIOSH).

Tilley, A.J., Wilkinson, R.T., Warren, P.S.G., Watson, B. and Drud, M. (1982) The sleep and performance of shift workers. *Hum. Factors*, **24**, 629–641.

Van Cauter, E. and Turek, F.W. (1990) Strategies for resetting the human circadian clock. *N. Engl. J. Med.*, **322**(18), 1306–1308.

Van Loon, J.H. (1963) Diurnal body temperature curves in shift workers. *Ergonomics*, **6**, 267–272.

Wever, R.A. (1979) *The Circadian System of Man: Results of Experiments Under Temporal Isolation*, New York: Springer-Verlag.

Wever, R.A. (1988) Order and disorder in human circadian rhythmicity: Possible relations to mental disorders. In *Biological Rhythms and Mental Disorders*, edited by Kupfer, D.J., Monk, T.H. and Barchas, J.D., pp. 238–324, New York: Guilford Press.

Williamson, A.M. and Sanderson, J.W. (1986) Changing the speed of shift rotation: A field study. *Ergonomics*, **29**, 1085–1096.

Chapter 10

Epilogue

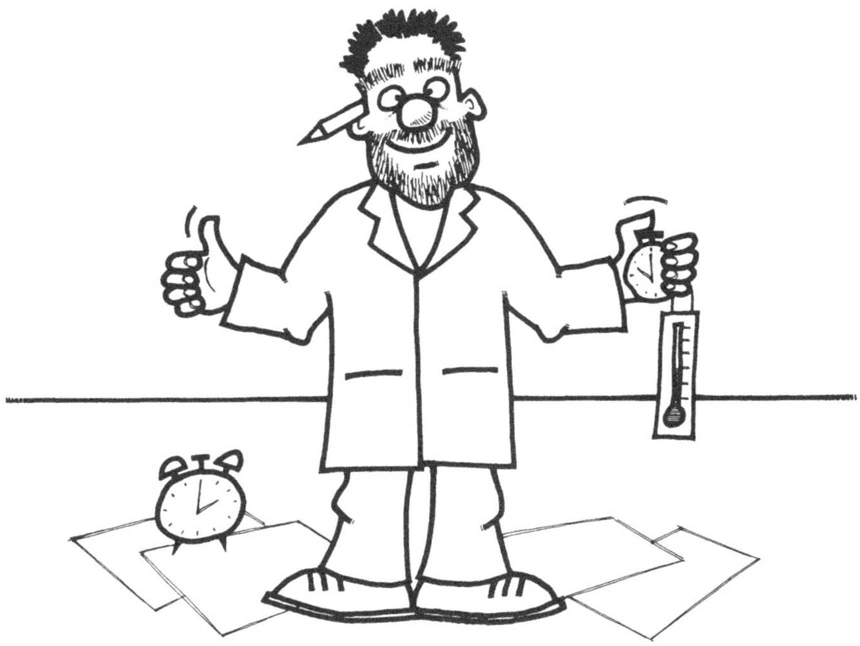

Like that of sleep research, the history of chronobiology is a relatively short one. Many of the original pioneers of chronobiology are still alive and active. The first task that faced these researchers was to convince a sceptical scientific establishment that the concept of homoeostatis did not rule supreme, that homoeostatic mechanisms produced rhythms rather than a fixed 'set point', and that the temporal structure of life was as important as its anatomical structure. It was an uphill struggle to convince their scientific colleagues that the circadian rhythms they observed were neither trivial nor artefactual. Although there are still a few pockets of resistance, this struggle has been largely won. In the main, even if not properly accounted for, circadian principles are certainly not derided as foolish (as they once were) and usually have at least 'lip service' paid to them.

Sadly, in the work setting, there is still a long way to go before circadian principles are adequately taken into account. Legislators and regulators (particularly in the UK and USA) have hardly begun to realize that an off-duty break at one time of day may be far less restorative than that at another. Only the more enlightened of legislative bodies and regulative agencies have directly addressed this issue, and even fewer have supported that approach with directly funded research. A major impediment to North American shift work research is that much of it has been conducted for profit while little of it has been published in respectable journals.

Employers, too, cannot escape without blame. While Henry Ford's production line has undoubtedly produced many material benefits to mankind (few could afford a hand-made car) there has been a huge cost in terms of the dehumanization of the employees involved. One aspect of that dehumanization is the false assumption that, like machines, human beings can perform just as well in the middle of the night as they can during the day. Although a shift differential is paid, this is viewed simply as recompense for a little discomfort, rather than anything more profound. Indeed, a senior manager of a large tyre manufacturer recently dismissed a researcher's concerns about shift work with the comment that 'We pay them enough to put up with a little inconvenience'.

Part of the reason for this neglect of circadian principles in the workplace has been a variant of the 'blame the victim' argument. In this approach the shift worker who cannot cope (and who is thus tardy, absent, unproductive or accident-prone) is blamed for not doing the right thing (i.e. not obtaining a full 8 hours of sleep during the day and not appearing for a night of work all 'bright-eyed and bushy-tailed'). This blame can either be dressed up as indolence or as an 'illness' (e.g. a medical sleep disorder), but in either case the employee, not the employer, is blamed. The shift worker then has the duty either to improve his efforts, seek medical assistance or resign from the job. The fact that it is perfectly natural for human beings to find night work difficult to cope with is conveniently ignored by most employers. Given that few, if any, organizations actually do anything to help their shift working employees to cope, this is inherently a rather unreasonable attitude for the employer to take. Using an analogy, everyone would ridicule a frozen food company that failed to provide protective gloves and clothing for its cold room workers, and then complained when they shivered, dropped things or stayed out in the warm. Is it really that unreasonable to expect night shift employers to provide an equivalent level of protection for their workforce?

Blame must not be placed solely upon the legislators and the employers, however. Shift workers are often their own worst enemy, resisting improvements to their shift systems and overburdening themselves with overtime, moonlighting jobs and other commitments. Very often the workers themselves adopt the attitude of 'Pay me a bit more money and all will be well'.

There are several areas, nowadays, where employers and employees have combined forces to promote programmes designed to make the workforce happier, safer and more productive. Most notable of these have been in the areas of smoking, fitness and drug and alcohol abuse. We feel very strongly that shift work coping should now be added to that list.

The decade of the 1990s may herald a crisis in terms of shift work coping ability. As we have discussed earlier, many shift workers start to have problems when they are middle aged and by the end of the 1990s most of the baby boom generation will be in their early to mid-fifties. Thus, there may prove to be too few people able to cope with the ever increasing shift work requirement stemming from expensive plant machinery and an increasing service sector. Before that crisis is reached, it is vital that all those concerned, the legislators, the employers and the employees, come to recognize the importance of the biological clock. The melatonin circulating in the bloodstream of an unadjusted night worker may be as much of a safety and health risk as the alcohol in the bloodstream of an inebriated dayworker!

Glossary

(This glossary is largely based on that in the US Congress: Office of Technology Assessment's 'Biological Rhythms: Implications for the worker' to which the reader is referred for further details (see Suggested further reading).

Afternoon shift: See *evening shift.*
Amplitude: As it relates to circadian rhythms, the difference between the maximum or minimum and mean values of a function (e.g. body temperature) during the circadian cycle. Amplitude provides a measure of extent of the fluctuation within a cycle.

Biological rhythm: A self-sustained, cyclic change in a physiological process or behavioural function that repeats at regular intervals. See *circadian rhythm, infradian rhythm, ultradian rhythm*.
Biorhythm theory: A theory that postulates three infradian rhythms that control human behaviour and performance. It has no scientific basis.
Body clock: The internal mechanism of the body that controls biological rhythms. See *circadian pacemaker*.
Bright light: Bright light has been shown to shift circadian rhythms and has been used to treat some sleep disorders and jet lag. In order to affect circadian rhythms it needs to have an intensity of at least 2 500 lux, which is equivalent to outdoor light at dawn.

Chronobiology: The scientific study of the effect of time on living systems, including the study of biological rhythms.
Circadian clock: See *circadian pacemaker*.
Circadian cycle: The 24-hour interval between recurrences of a defined phase of a circadian rhythm. See *circadian rhythm*.
Circadian pacemaker: An internal timekeeping mechanism capable of driving or co-ordinating circadian rhythms. See *circadian rhythm, suprachiasmatic nucleus*.
Circadian rhythm: A self-sustained biological rhythm which in a natural environment is normally synchronized to a 24-hour period. See *biological rhythm*.
Circadian rhythm desynchronization: See *circadian rhythm disruption*.
Circadian rhythm disruption: Disorganization among circadian rhythms or desynchrony between body clock generated rhythms and the 24-hour cycle in the environment.
Clockwise shift rotation: A work schedule in which the shifts move forward (i.e. delay) from day to evening to night. See *rotating shift*, compare *counterclockwise shift rotation*.
Compressed workweek: A schedule in which employees work approximately 40 hours in fewer than 5 days.

Cortisol: A steroid hormone secreted by humans; cortisol secretion exhibits a circadian rhythm and is used as a marker for the body's pacemaker.
Counterclockwise shift rotation: A work schedule in which the shifts move backward (i.e. advance), from night to evening to day. See *rotating shift*; compare *clockwise shift rotation*.
Current Population Survey: A survey of 55 000 to 60 000 sample households conducted monthly by the Bureau of the Census for the Bureau of Labor Statistics (USA). Supplements to the survey have incorporated questions on shift work.

Day shift: As defined in Current Population Surveys, a period of work in which half or more of the hours worked are between 8 am and 4 pm.
Diurnal: Being active during the day.
Double shift: Two consecutive shifts worked in a single 24-hour period.

Entraining agent (or Zeitgeber): A factor that synchronizes an organism's biological rhythms to the outside world; for example, the light-dark cycle is an entraining agent for circadian rhythms.
Environmental cue: A signal from outside an organism that prompts it to some action.
Evening person: A general term used to describe an individual who has difficulty waking up, is able to sleep late in the morning, and finds it difficult to fall asleep at night. Compare *morning person*.
Evening (or afternoon) shift: As defined by the Current Population Survey, a period of work in which half or more of the hours worked are between 4 pm and midnight.
Extended duty hours: Long periods of work (usually over 12 hours) that may cause a worker to get less than the usual amount of sleep.

Fatigue: Weariness caused by physical and mental exertion.
Field study: Used in this book to refer to an investigation in which a researcher observes workers in their actual work environment and on their actual shift system. Compare *laboratory study, survey study*.
Fixed (or permanent) shift: A work schedule in which the hours of work remain the same from day to day. Compare *rotating shift, irregular shift*.
Flexitime: A system in which the starting and finishing times of a shift or period of duty are determined by the individual worker, with a required number of total hours specified by the employer. Usually there is a daily core period when all workers must be present.
Free-running rhythm: A circadian rhythm operating in the absence of environmental cues; such rhythms may be 20 to 28 hours in length. Under free-running conditions, the human body clock has a circadian rhythm of about 25 hours.
Full-time employment: A job requiring 35 or more hours of work per week. Compare *part-time employment, shortened workweek*.

Infradian rhythm: A biological rhythm with a cycle of more than 24 hours; for example, the human menstrual cycle. See *biological rhythm*; compare *ultradian rhythm*.
Internal clock: See *circadian pacemaker*.
Internal desynchronization: Loss of synchronization among rhythms within a single organism.

Irregular shift: A work schedule that is variable and erratic. Compare *fixed shift, rotating shift*.

Jet lag: The malaise associated with travel across time zones; it results from conflict between the traveller's internal clock and the external rhythms in the new time zone.

Laboratory study: Used in this book to refer to an investigation in which the researcher attempts to simulate the shift system and workplace in a controlled environment. Compare *field study, survey study*.

Longitudinal study: Analysis of a function in the same experimental subjects over a period of time; especially useful in determining effects that vary widely among individuals.

Melatonin: A hormone produced by the pineal gland, which is present in many animals, including humans. Melatonin secretion is circadian, and production is readily inhibited by light. Melatonin is being investigated as a possible circadian entraining agent in humans. See *entraining agent*.

Microsleep: Brief episode of sleep experienced by a person who is so tired that he or she cannot resist sleep.

Moonlighting: Holding more than one paid job.

Morning person: A general term used to describe an individual who wakes up easily, has difficulty sleeping in late, and falls asleep quickly at night. Compare *evening person*.

Night shift: As defined in the Current Population Survey, a period of work in which half or more of the hours worked are between midnight and 8 am.

Night shift paralysis: A rare condition marked by short-term paralysis, usually lasting about two minutes, during which individuals are aware of their surroundings but are unable to move; it is associated with extreme sleep deprivation.

Nocturnal: Being active at night.

Non-REM sleep: The four stages of sleep during which the sleeper does not experience rapid eye movement (REM) sleep. See *slow wave sleep, rapid eye movement (REM) sleep*.

Overtime: Time worked at one job in excess of the contracted (e.g. 40) hours per week. Overtime may be required or voluntary.

Part-time employment: A job consisting of fewer than 35 hours of work per week. Compare *full-time employment, shortened workweek*.

Permanent shift: See *fixed shift*.

Phase shift: The resetting of an organism's internal clock in response to an entraining agent. The organism's circadian rhythms may be advanced, delayed, or not shifted at all, depending on the timing of exposure. See *entraining agent*.

Rapid eye movement (REM) sleep: Stage of sleep during which the eyes move rapidly and brain activity resembles that observed during wakefulness. Heart rate and respiration increase and become erratic, and vivid dreams are frequent. REM sleep alternates with non-REM sleep in ultradian cycles lasting 90 to 100 minutes. Compare *slow wave sleep*.

Rotating shift: Work in which the hours change regularly, for example from a day to an evening to a night shift. Rotation may be rapid (e.g. 3 days), mid length (e.g. 1 week), or long (e.g. 4 weeks); and may be forward or backward (see above). Compare *fixed shift, irregular shift*.

Shift maladaptation syndrome: A combination of ailments arising from the inability of some workers to adjust to long-term shift work.

Shiftwork: Used in this book to refer to any nonstandard work schedule (including evening or night shifts, rotating shifts, split shifts, and extended duty hours) in which hours are commonly or always worked outside the period between 7 am and 6 pm. See *day shift, evening shift, night shift, rotating shift, split shift, extended duty hours*.

Shift worker: A person who works a nonstandard schedule. See *shiftwork*.

Shortened workweek: A schedule of full-time employment that entails 35 or fewer hours of work per week.

Sleep debt: The state of chronic fatigue and sleepiness that may result from the lack of sufficient sleep or disrupted sleep. See *fatigue, sleep deprivation*.

Sleep deprivation: Lack of sufficient sleep. Compare *fatigue*.

Slow wave sleep: The stages of sleep during which the eyes do not move, heart rate and respiration are slow and steady, muscles show little movement, and dreams are infrequent. Compare *rapid eye movement (REM) sleep*.

Split shift: A schedule of full-time work in which a period of work is followed by a break and then another period of work.

Stressor: Any source of stress. Used in this book primarily to refer to the disruption of circadian rhythms, the disruption of sleep, and the social and domestic disturbances caused by shift work.

Subjective day: The portion of an organism's internal cycle that normally occurs during the day.

Subjective night: The portion of an organism's internal cycle that normally occurs during the night.

Suprachiasmatic nucleus: A region of the brain of mammals that acts as an organism's primary circadian pacemaker, controlling or co-ordinating its circadian rhythms. See *circadian pacemaker*.

Survey study: Used in this book to refer to an investigation in which the researcher asks the worker questions and elicits answers, usually in one or two interviews or classroom-like sessions. Survey studies are often conducted before and after an intervention in order to gauge its impact. Compare *field study, laboratory study*.

Transmeridian flight: Travel across time zones. See *jet lag*.

Ultradian rhythm: A biological rhythm with a cycle of less than 24 hours; human sleep cycles and the release of some hormones are examples. See *biological rhythm*; compare *infradian rhythm*.

Weekend shift: A work schedule in which a separate workforce is used to work 12 hours per day, 2 days per week.

Zeitgeber: See *Entraining agent*.

Suggested further reading

Costa, G., Cesana, G., Kogi, K. and Wedderburn, A. (Eds) (1990) *Shiftwork: Health, Sleep and Performance*, Frankfurt am Main: Peter Lang.

Folkard, S. (Ed.) (1987) Irregular and abnormal hours of work. *Ergonomics*, **30** (Special issue).

Folkard, S. and Monk, T.H. (Eds) (1985) *Hours of Work: Temporal Factors in Work Scheduling*, Chichester: J. Wiley & Sons.

Haider, M., Koller, M. and Cervinka, R. (Eds) (1986) *Night and Shiftwork: Longterm Effects and their Prevention*, Frankfurt am Main: Peter Lang.

Johnson, L.C., Tepas, D.I., Colquhoun, W.P. and Colligan, M.J. (Eds) (1981) *Biological Rhythms, Sleep and Shift Work*, New York: Spectrum Publications.

Kogi, K., Miura, T. and Saito, H. (Eds) (1982) Shiftwork: its practice and improvement. *Journal of Human Ergology*, **11** (supplement).

Monk, T.H. (1988) *How to Make Shiftwork Safe and Productive*, American Society of Safety Engineers: Des Plaines, Ill.

Monk, T.H. (Ed) (1991) *Sleeps, Sleepiness and Performance*, Chichester: J. Wiley & Sons.

Oginski, A., Pokorski, J. and Rutenfranz, J. (Eds) (1987) *Contemporary Advances in Shiftwork Research*, Krakow: Medical Academy.

Reinberg, A., Vieux, N. and Andlauer, P. (Eds) (1981) *Night and Shift Work: Biological and Social Aspects*, Oxford: Pergamon Press.

Scott, A.J. (Ed.) (1990) *Shiftwork. State of the art reviews in Occupational Medicine*, Vol 5, Philadelphia: Hanley & Belfus, Inc.

US Congress: Office of Technology Assessment (1991) *Biological Rhythms: Implications for the Worker*. OTA-BA-463, U.S. Government Printing Office: Washington DC.

Bibliography

Adams, J., Folkard, S. and Young, M. (1986) Coping strategies used by nurses on night duty. *Ergonomics*, **29**, 185–196.

Akerstedt, T. (1985) Shifted sleep hours. *Ann. Clin. Res.*, **17**, 273–279.

Akerstedt, T. (1988) Sleepiness as a consequence of shift work. *Sleep*, **11**, 17–34.

Akerstedt, T. and Froberg, J. (1976) Shift work and health-interdisciplinary aspects. In *Shift Work and Health, HEW Publication No. (NIOSH) 76–203*, edited by Rentos, P.G. and Shepard, R.D. (Washington, DC: US Department of Health, Education and Welfare), pp. 179–197.

Akerstedt, T. and Gillberg, M. (1981) The circadian variation of experimentally displaced sleep. *Sleep*, **4**, 159–169.

Akerstedt, T., Gillberg, M. and Wetterberg, L. (1982) The circadian covariation of fatigue and urinary melatonin. *Biol. Psychiatry*, **17**, 547–552.

Akerstedt, T. and Levi, L. (1978) Circadian rhythms in the secretion of cortisol, adrenalin and noradrenalin. *Eur. J. Clin. Invest.*, **8**, 57–58.

Akerstedt, T., Patkai, P. and Dahlgren, K. (1977) Field studies of shiftwork: II. Temporal patterns in psychophysiological activation in workers alternating between night and day work. *Ergonomics*, **20**, 621–631.

Akerstedt, T. and Torsvall, L. (1978) Experimental changes in shift schedules – Their effects on well-being. *Ergonomics*, **21**, 849–856.

Akerstedt, T., Torsvall, L. and Gillberg, M. (1987) Sleepiness in shiftwork: A review with emphasis on continuous monitoring of EEG and EOG. *Chronobiol. Int.*, **4**, 129–140.

Anderson, R.M., Jr. and Bremer, D. (1987) Sleep duration at home and sleepiness on the job in rotating twelve-hour shift workers. *Hum. Factors*, **29**, 477–481.

Angersbach, D., Knauth, P., Loskant, H., Karvonen, M.J., Undeutsch, K. and Rutenfranz, J. (1980) A retrospective cohort study comparing complaints and diseases in day and shift workers. *Int. Arch. Occup. Environ. Health*, **45**, 127–140.

Ansseau, M., Kupfer, D.J., Reynolds, C.F. and McEachran, A.B. (1984) REM latency distribution in major depression: Clinical characteristics associated with sleep onset REM periods. *Biol. Psychiatry*, **19**, 1651–1666.

Aschoff, J. (1978) Features of circadian rhythms relevant for the design of shift schedules. *Ergonomics*, **21**, 739–755.

Casale, G., Butte, M., Pasotti, C., Ravecca, D. and DeNicola, P. (1983) Antithrombin III and circadian rhythms in the aged and in myocardial infarction. *Haematologica*, **68**, 615–619.

Colligan, M.J. and Tepas, D.I. (1986) The stress of hours of work. *Am. Ind. Hyg. Assoc. J.*, **47**, 686–695.

Colquhoun, W.P. (1976) Psychological and psychophysiological aspects of work and fatigue. *Act. Nerv. Super.*, **18**, 257–263.

Colquhoun, W.P. (1976) Accidents, injuries and shift work. In *Shift Work and Health*, HEW Publication No. (NIOSH) 76–203, edited by Rentos, P.G. and Shepard, R.D., pp. 160–175. Washington, DC: US Department of Health, Education and Welfare.

Colquhoun, W.P., Blake, M.J.F. and Edwards, R.S. (1968) Experimental studies of shift work II: Stabilized 8 hour shift systems. *Ergonomics*, **11**, 527–546.

Colquhoun, W.P., Blake, M.J.F. and Edwards, R.S. (1968) Experimental studies of shift work I: A comparison of 'rotating' and 'stabilized' 4 hour shift systems. *Ergonomics*, **11**, 437–453.

Colquhoun, W.P., Blake, M.J.F. and Edwards, R.S. (1969) Experimental studies of shift work III: Stabilized 12 hour shift systems. *Ergonomics*, **12**, 865–882.

Colquhoun, W.P. and Edwards, R.S. (1970) Circadian rhythms of body temperature in shift workers at a coalface. *Br. J. Ind. Med.*, **27**, 266–272.

Colquhoun, W.P. and Folkard, S. (1978) Personality differences in body-temperature rhythm, and their relation to its adjustment to night work. *Ergonomics*, **21**, 811–817.

Conroy, R.T.W.L., Elliott, A.L. and Mills, J.N. (1970) Circadian excretory rhythms in night workers. *Br. J. Ind. Med.*, **27**, 356–363.

Costa, G., Gaffuri, E., Perfranceschi, G. and Tarsella, M. (1979) Re-entrainment of diurnal variation of psychological and physiological performance at the end of a slowly rotated shift system in hospital workers. *Int. Arch. Occup. Environ. Health*, **44**, 165–175.

Craik, F.I.M. and Blankstein, K.R. (1975) Psychophysiology and human memory. In: *Research in Psychophysiology*, edited by Venables, P.H. and Christie, M.J., pp. 388–417. London: Wiley.

Czeisler, C.A., Kronauer, R.W., Allan, J.S. *et al.* (1989) Bright light induction of strong (Type 0) resetting of the human circadian pacemaker. *Science*, **244**, 1328–1333.

Czeisler, C.A., Moore-Ede, M.C. and Coleman, R.M. (1982) Rotating shift work schedules that disrupt sleep are improved by applying circadian principles. *Science*, **217**, 460–463.

Dahlgren, K. (1981) Temporal patterns in psychophysiological activation in rotating shift workers – A follow-up field study one year after an increase in night time work. *Scand. J. Work Environ. Health*, **7**, 131–140.

Dahlgren, K. (1981) Adjustment of circadian rhythms and EEG sleep functions to day and night sleep among permanent and rotating shift-workers. *Psychophysiology*, **18**, 381–391.

Dahlgren, K. (1981) Long-term adjustment of circadian rhythms to a rotating shiftwork schedule. *Scand. J. Work Environ. Health*, **7**, 141–151.

DeVries-Griever, A.H.G. and Meijman, T.F. (1987) The impact of abnormal hours of work on various modes of information processing: A process model on human costs of performance. *Ergonomics*, **30**, 1287–1299.

Eastman, C.I. (1987) Bright light in work–sleep schedules for shift workers: Application of circadian rhythm principles. In *Temporal Disorder in Human Oscillatory Systems*, edited by Rensing, L., Van der Heiden, U. and Mackey, M.C. (New York: Springer-Verlag), pp. 176–185.

Fischer, F.M. (1986) Retrospective study regarding absenteeism among shiftworkers. *Int. Arch. Occup. Environ. Health*, **58**, 301–320.

Fischer, F.M. *et al.* (1989) Biological aspects and self evaluation of shiftwork adaptation. *Int. Arch. Occ. Environ. Health*, **61**, 379–384.

Fisher, M., Rutishau, I.H. and Read, R.S.D. (1986) The dietary patterns of shiftworkers on short rotation shifts. *Community Health Stud.*, **10**, 54–56.

Folkard, S. (1986) Our diurnal nature. *Br. Med. J.*, **293**, 1257–1258.

Folkard, S. and Condon, R. (1987) Night shift paralysis in air traffic control officers. *Ergonomics*, **30**, 1353–1363.

Folkard, S., Knauth, P., Monk, T.H. and Rutenfranz, J. (1976) The effect of memory load on the circadian variation in performance efficiency under a rapidly rotating shift system. *Ergonomics*, **19**, 479–488.

Folkard, S. and Monk, T.H. (1981) Individual differences in the circadian response to a weekly rotating shift system. In *Night and Shift Work: Biological and Social Aspects*, edited by Reinberg, A., Vieux, N. and Andlauer, P., pp. 365–374, Oxford: Pergamon Press.

Folkard, S., Monk, T.H. and Lobban, M.C. (1978) Short and long-term adjustment of circadian rhythms in 'permanent' night nurses. *Ergonomics*, **21**, 785–799.

Folkard, S., Monk, T.H. and Lobban, M.C. (1979) Towards a predictive test of adjustment to shiftwork. *Ergonomics*, **22**, 79–91.

Foret, J. and Benoit, O. (1980) Predictable effects on individual sleep patterns during a rapidly rotating shift system. *Int. Arch. Occup. Environ. Health.*, **45**, 49–56.

Foret, J., Bensimon, G., Benoit, O. and Vieux, N. (1981) Quality of sleep as a function of age and shift work. In *Night and Shift Work:*

Biological and Social Aspects, edited by Reinberg, A., Vieux, N. and Andlauer, P., pp. 149–160. Oxford: Pergamon Press.

Frese, M. and Okonek, K. (1984) Reasons to leave shiftwork and psychological and psychosomatic complaints of former shiftworkers. *J. Appl. Psychol.*, **69**, 509–514.

Friedman, R.C., Bigger, J.T. and Kornfeld, D.S. (1971) The intern and sleep loss. *N. Engl. J. Med.*, **285**, 201–203.

Gadbois, C. (1981) Women on night shift: Interdependence of sleep and off-the-job activities. In *Night and Shift Work: Biological and Social Aspects*, edited by Reinberg, A., Vieux, N. and Andlauer, P., pp. 223–227, Oxford: Pergamon Press.

Gordon, N.P., Cleary, P.D., Parker, C.E. and Czeisler, C.A. (1985) Sleeping pill use, heavy drinking and other unhealthful practices and consequences associated with shift work: A national probability sample study. *Sleep Res.*, **14**, 94.

Gordon, N.P., Cleary, P.D., Parker, C.E. and Czeisler, C.A. (1986) The prevalence and health impact of shiftwork. *Am. J. Public Health*, **76**, 1225–1228.

Harma, M.I., Ilmarinen, J., Knauth, P., Rutenfranz, J. and Hanninen, O. (1988) Physical training intervention in female shift workers: I. The effects of intervention on fitness, fatigue, sleep and psychosomatic symptoms. *Ergonomics*, **31**, 51–63.

Harrington, J.M. (1978) *Shiftwork and Health. A Critical Review of the Literature*, London: HMSO.

Hedman, B.K. and Swensson, A. (1975) Problems related to shift work: a field study of Swedish railroad workers with irregular work hours. *Scand. J. Work Environ. Health*, **1**, 254–262.

Hildebrandt, G. (1986) Individual differences in susceptibility to night- and shift work. In *Night and Shiftwork: Long term Effects and their Prevention*, edited by Haider, M., Koller, M. and Cervinka, R., pp. 109–116, Peter Lang: Frankfurt am Main.

Hildebrandt, G. and Stratmann, I. (1979) Circadian system response to night work in relation to the individual circadian phase position. *Int. Arch. Occup. Environ. Health*, **43**, 73–83.

Khaleque, A. (1984) Circadian rhythms in heart rate of shift and day workers. *J. Hum. Ergol.*, **13**, 23–29.

Knauth, P. and Kiesswetter, E. (1987) A change from weekly to quicker shift rotations: A field study of discontinuous three-shift workers. *Ergonomics*, **30**, 1311–1321.

Knauth, P., Landau, K., Droge, C., Schwitteck, M., Widynski, M. and Rutenfranz, J. (1980) Duration of sleep depending on the type of shift work. *Int. Arch. Occup. Environ. Health*, **46**, 167–177.

Knauth, P. and Rutenfranz, J. (1976) Circadian rhythm of body temperature and re-entrainment at shift change. *Int. Arch. Occup. Environ. Health*, **37**, 125–137.

Knauth, P., Rutenfranz, J. Hermann, G. and Poppl, S.J. (1978) Re-entrainment of physiological functions in experimental shiftwork studies. *Ergonomics*, **21**, 775–783.

Knutsson, A., Akerstedt, T. and Orth-Gomer, K. (1986) Increased risk of ischaemic heart disease in shift workers. *Lancet*, **12**, 89–92.

Koller, M., Kundi, M. and Cervinka, R. (1978) Field studies of shiftwork at an Austrian oil refinery. I: Health and psychosocial well-being of workers who drop out of shiftwork. *Ergonomics*, **21**, 835–847.

Kolmodin-Hedman, B. and Swensson, A. (1975) Problems related to shift work: a field study of Swedish railroad workers with irregular work hours. *Scand. J. Work, Environ. Health*, **1**, 254–262.

Lortie, M., Foret, J., Teiger, C. and Laville, A. (1979) Circadian rhythms and behavior of permanent nightworkers. *Int. Arch. Occup. Environ. Health*, **44**, 1–11.

Meers, A., Maasen, A. and Verhaegen, P. (1978) Subjective health after six months and after four years of shift work. *Ergonomics*, **21**, 857–861.

Melbin, M. (1978) Night as frontier. *Am. Sociol. Rev.*, **43**, 2–22.

Mills, J.N., Minors, D.S. and Waterhouse, J.M. (1978) Adaptation to abrupt time shifts of the oscillator(s) controlling human circadian rhythms. *J. Physiol.*, **285**, 455–470.

Minors, D.S. and Waterhouse, J.M. (1988) Effects upon circadian rhythmicity of an alteration to the sleep–wake cycle: Problems of assessment resulting from measurement in the presence of sleep and analysis in terms of a single shifted component. *J. Biol. Rhythms*, **3**, 23–40.

Monk, T.H. (1986) Advantages and disadvantages of rapidly rotating shift schedules – A circadian viewpoint. *Hum. Factors*, **28**, 553–557.

Monk, T.H. and Embrey, D.E. (1981) A field study of circadian rhythms in actual and interpolated task performance. In *Night and Shift Work: Biological and Social Aspects*, edited by Reinberg, A., Vieux, N. and Andlauer, P., pp. 473–480, Oxford: Pergamon Press.

Monk, T.H. and Folkard, S. (1983) Circadian rhythms and shiftwork. In *Stress and Fatigue in Human Performance*, edited by Hockey, G.R.J., pp. 97–121, New York: John Wiley & Sons.

Moog, R. (1987) Optimization of shift work: Physiological contributions. *Ergonomics*, **30**, 1249–1259.

Moog, R. and Hildebrandt, G. (1987) Circadian adaptation to fast and slow rotating shift systems. *Prog. Clin. Biol. Res.*, **227B**, 403–414.

Moore-Ede, M.C. and Richardson, G.S. (1985) Medical implications of shiftwork. *Annu. Rev. Med.*, **36**, 607–617.

Orth-Gomer, K. (1983) Intervention on coronary risk factors by adapting a shift work schedule to biologic rhythmicity. *Psychosom. Med.*, **45**, 407–415.

Patkai, P., Akerstedt, T. and Pettersson, K. (1977) Field studies of shiftwork I: Temporal patterns in psychophysiological activation in permanent night workers. *Ergonomics*, **20**, 611–619.

Reinberg, A., Andlauer, P., DePrins, J., Malbecq, W., Vieux, N. and Bourdeleau, P. (1984) Desynchronization of the oral temperature circadian rhythm and intolerance to shift work. *Nature*, **308**, 272–274.

Reinberg, A., Smolensky, M. and Labrecque, G. (1987) The hunting of a wonder pill for resetting all biological clocks. *Annu. Rev. Chronopharmacol.*, **4**, 171–208.

Reinberg, A., Motohashi, Y., Bourdeleau, P., Andlauer, P., Levi, F. and Bicakova-Rocher, A. (1988) Alteration of period and amplitude of circadian rhythms in shift workers with special reference to temperature, right and left hand grip strength. *Eur. J. Appl. Physiol.*, **57**, 15–25.

Rutenfranz, J., Knauth, P. and Colquhoun, W.P. (1976) Hours of work and shiftwork. *Ergonomics*, **19**, 331–340.

Rutenfranz, J., Colquhoun, W.P., Knauth, P. and Ghata, J.N. (1977) Biomedical and psychosocial aspects of shift work: A review. *Scand. J. Work Environ. Health*, **3**, 165–182.

Scherrer, J. (1981) Man's work and circadian rhythm through the ages. In *Night and Shift Work: Biological and Social Aspects*, edited by Reinberg, A., Vieux, N. and Andlauer, P., pp. 1–10, Oxford: Pergamon Press.

Schwarzenau, P., Knauth, P., Kiesswetter, E., Brockmann, W. and Rutenfranz, J. (1986) Algorithms for the computerized construction of shift systems which meet ergonomic criteria. *Appl. Ergonomics*, **17**, 169–176.

Shift Work Committee: Japan Association of Industrial Health (1979) Opinion on night work and shift work. *J. Science Labour*, **55**, 1–36 (Abstract).

Smith, A. and Miles, C. (1986) Acute effects of meals, noise and nightwork. *Br. J. Psychol.*, **77**, 377–387.

Smith, P.A. (1979) A study of weekly and rapidly rotating shiftworkers. *Int. Arch. Occup. Environ. Health*, **43**, 211–220 (Abstract).

Tarquini, B., Cecchettin, M. and Cariddi, A. (1986) Serum gastrin and pepsinogen in shift workers. *Int. Arch. Occup. Environ. Health*, **58**, 99–103.

Taylor, P.J. and Pocock, S.J. (1972) Mortality of shift and day workers 1956–1968. *Br. J. Ind. Med.*, **29**, 201–207.

Tepas, D.I. and Mahan, R.P. (1989) The many meanings of sleep. *Work and Stress*, **3**, 93–102.

Torsvall, L. and Akerstedt, T. (1980) A diurnal type scale: Construction, consistency, and validation in shift work. *Scand. J. Work Environ. Health*, **6**, 283–290.

Van Loon, J.H. (1963) Diurnal body temperature curves in shift workers. *Ergonomics*, **6**, 267–272.

Verhaegen, P., Maasen, A. and Meers, A. (1982) Health problems in shift workers. In *Biological Rhythms and Shift Work*, edited by Johnson, L.C., Tepas, D.I., Colquhoun, W.P. and Colligan, M.J., pp. 271–282, New York: Spectrum.

Vidacek, S., Kaliterna, L. and Folkard, S. (1986) Productivity on a weekly rotating shift system: Circadian adjustment and sleep deprivation effects? *Ergonomics*, **29**, 1583–1590.

Vokac, Z., Magnus, P.M., Jebens, E. and Gundersen, N. (1981) Apparent phase-shifts of circadian rhythms (masking effects) during rapid shift rotation. *Int. Arch. Occup. Environ. Health*, **49**, 53–65.

Waldhauser, F., Vierhapper, H. and Pirich, K. (1986) Abnormal circadian melatonin secretion in night-shift workers. *N. Engl. J. Med.*, **315**, 1614.

Walker, J.M. (1978) *The Human Aspects of Shiftwork*, Bath: The Pitman Press.

Walsh, J.K., Muehlbach, M.J. and Schweitzer, P.K. (1984) Acute administration of triazolam for the daytime sleep of rotating shift workers. *Sleep*, **7**, 223–229.

Walsh, J.KJ., Sugerman, J.L., Muehlbach, M.J. and Schweitzer, P.K. (1988) Physiological sleep tendency on a simulated night shift: Adaptation and effects of triazolam. *Sleep*, **11**, 251–264.

Walsh, J.K., Tepas, D.I. and Moss, P.D. (1981) The EEG sleep of night and rotating shift workers. In *The Twenty-four Hour Workday: Proceedings of a Symposium on Variations in Work–Sleep Schedules*, edited by Johnson, L.C. Tepas, D.I., Colquhoun, W.P. and Colligan, M.J., pp. 451–465, Cincinnati, OH: Department of Health and Human Services (NIOSH).

Webb, W.B. and Agnew, H.W., Jr. (1978) Effects of rapidly rotating shifts on sleep patterns and sleep structure. *Aviation, Space and Environmental Medicine*, **49**, 384–389.

Wedderburn, A.A.I. (1967) Social factors in satisfaction with swiftly rotating shifts. *Occup. Psychol.*, **41**, 85–107.

Weitzman, E.D. and Kripke, D.F. (1981) Experimental 12-hour shift of the sleep–wake cycle in man: Effects on sleep and physiologic rhythms. In *Variations in Work–Sleep Schedules: Effects on Health and Performance, Advances in Sleep Research*, Volume 7, edited by Johnson, L.C., Tepas, D.I., Colquhoun, W.P. and Colligan, M.J., pp. 93–110, New York: Spectrum Publications.

Wilkinson, R.T. and Edwards, R.S. (1968) Stable hours and varied work as aids to efficiency. *Psychon. Sci.*, **13**, 205–206.

Williamson, A.M. and Sanderson, J.W. (1986) Changing the speed of shift rotation: A field study. *Ergonomics*, **29**, 1085–1096.

Wojtczak-Jaroszowa, J. and Jarosz, D. (1987) Chronohygienic and chronosocial aspects of industrial accidents. *Prog. Clin. Biol. Res.*, **227B**, 415–426.

Index